TREATMENT
AND
MANAGEMENT
OF OBESITY

Edited by

George A. Bray, M.D.

Professor of Medicine and
Director of the Clinical Research Center
Harbor General Hospital
U.C.L.A. Campus
Torrance, California

and

John E. Bethune, M.D.

Professor and Chairman
Department of Medicine
University of Southern California
School of Medicine
Los Angeles, California

TREATMENT
AND
MANAGEMENT
OF OBESITY

Medical Department
Harper & Row, Publishers
Hagerstown, Maryland
New York, Evanston, San Francisco, London

Standard Book Number: 06-140544-2
Library of Congress Catolog Card Number:
73-22122

Contents

III. NEWER APPROACHES TO THE TREATMENT OF OBESITY

Contributors

DAVID H. BLANKENHORN, M.D.
Professor of Medicine and Chief, Section of Cardiology, University of Southern California School of Medicine, Los Angeles, California (p. 77)

GEORGE A. BRAY, M.D.
Professor of Medicine and Director of the Clinical Research Center, Harbor General Hospital-U.C.L.A. Campus, Torrance, California (p. 61, 117)

GEORGE F. CAHILL, Jr., M.D.
Professor and Director of Medicine, Elliot P. Joslin Research Laboratory, Harvard Medical School, Boston, Massachusetts (p. 3)

LOREN T. DeWIND, M.D.
Assistant Clinical Professor of Medicine, University of Southern California School of Medicine, Los Angeles, California (p. 132)

GRANT GWINUP, M.D.
Professor of Medicine and Chairman, Division of Endocrinology and Metabolism, University of California School of Medicine, Irvine, California (p. 93)

RICHARD E. NISBETT, Ph.D.
Associate Professor of Psychology, University of Michigan, Ann Arbor, Michigan (p. 45)

DONALD W. PETIT, M.D.
Clinical Professor of Medicine, University of Southern California School of Medicine, Los Angeles, California (p. 84)

LESTER B. SALANS, M.D.
Associate Professor of Medicine, Dartmouth Medical School, Hanover, New Hampshire (p. 17)

ETHAN A. H. SIMS, M.D.
Professor of Medicine and Director of Metabolic Unit, University of Vermont, Burlington, Vermont (p. 28)

ALBERT J. STUNKARD, M.D.
Professor and Chairman, Department of Psychiatry, Stanford University Medical Center, Stanford, California (p. 103)

Preface

In the spring of 1972 the University of Southern California offered a postgraduate course to the medical community on "The Obese and Their Ills." The material presented by the various speakers at this course presented much of what is new concerning obesity. After careful deliberation, it was decided to make the proceedings available for the general medical public.

It might well be asked, "Why another book about obesity?" The answer was the need for an inexpensive yet authoritative volume covering all of the current aspects of the problem. There is a long and growing list of best-selling books in this field including such titles as *Dr. Atkins' Diet Revolution, The Quick Weight Loss Diet, The Truth About Weight Control,* and *Think Yourself Thin.* Alongside of this list of how-to-do-it books are the few that have provided a more introspective and in-depth look at the problem. Such books include *Obesity: Medical and Scientific Aspects* (1), *Obesity and Its Management* (2), *Overweight Causes, Cost and Control* (3), and *Slim Chance in a Fat World: Behavioral Control of Obesity* (4). Most of these, too, suffer from a lack of depth of presentation. Our approach as been to take the papers presented in Los Angeles in 1972, update them to early 1973, and then edit them for readability.

The approach taken is the presentation of chapters dealing with basic principles, followed by clinical investigations, and finally a discussion of therapeutic approaches. In the first section we discuss the problem of energy expenditure, the role of the size of the fat cell in the development and persistence of obesity, the consequences of overeating both to the endocrine or glandular system and to the function of the eating centers on the brain.

In the second section we examine the kinds of obesity that are known and the way obesity influences the medical history of the patient.

In the final section we turn to therapy. There have been sigificant therapeutic advances toward several aspects of the problem. The role of exercise and diet are dealt with first. Clearly the most important adjunct to diet therapy has been the use of techniques of behavior modification, which are clearly spelled out. Pharmacological agents as adjuncts in the treatment of obesity are on the threshold of major new breakthroughs. Finally, the use of certain forms of surgery has had a great deal to offer to those patients who are afflicted with an overwhelming problem which has not been treatable by other means.

On the whole the book is aimed at providing answers to the questions about the development of obesity, but it is also helpful in its outlook toward the successful treatment of patients with obesity.

REFERENCES

1. Baird IM, Howard AN: Obesity: Medical and Scientific Aspects. Livingstone, Edinburgh, 1969.
2. Craddock D: Obesity and Its Management. Livingstone, Edinburgh, 1969.
3. Mayer J: Overweight Causes, Cost and Control. Prentice-Hall, Englewood Cliffs, NJ, 1968
4. Stuart RB, Davis B: Slim Chance in a Fat World: Behavioral Control of Obesity. Research Press, Champaigne, Ill. 1972

PATHOPHYSIOLOGY OF OBESITY

I

Obesity and the Control of Fuel Metabolism

1

GEORGE F. CAHILL, JR.

In the presence of oxygen, energy inherent in the carbon-hydrogen bond will be released. Whether this occurs by lighting the cooking gas on the stove—*i.e.,* by burning methane or propane—or whether it occurs from starting the engine of an automobile or by metabolizing substrates in the body, it is precisely the same chemical process. Plants, on the other hand, contain chlorophyll which can take the energy from sunlight and, in the presence of water and carbon dioxide, resynthesize carbon-hydrogen bonds.

Two kinds of carbon-hydrogen bonds constitute the way that nature can store energy. One is the basic structure of fat with two hydrogen atoms per carbon atom, and the other is in the form of compounds that substitute a hydroxyl group for one of the hydrogens. The latter is the basic structure of carbohydrate (Fig. 1-1). Examination of these two formulas reveals that carbohydrate obviously has available only one potentially oxidizable carbon-hydrogen bond. Therefore, on a per-carbon basis, carbohydrate will yield only half the energy that fat will yield. That is, fat has two hydrogens potentially available for oxidation, whereas

3

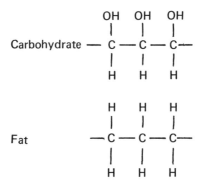

Fig. 1-1. Differences between chemical structures of carbohydrates and fats. Each carbohydrate carbon (*top*) contains a hydroxyl group and is thus more oxidized than the corresponding hydrogen–carbon atom in the fatty acid molecule (*bottom*). Because of this partial oxidation of the carbohydrate molecule, there are more calories per gram of fat than per gram of carbohydrate.

carbohydrate has only one. Indeed, the nutritionists tell us that fat as triglyceride yields a theoretical 9.4 Cal/g, whereas carbohydrate yields only about 4 cal/g, as apparent in Figure 1-1.

When plants became animals and had to carry their energy stores with them, fat synthesis obviously became paramount to survival, because it was a more economical form in which to transport energy. This is particularly true if one has to work against gravity. One might, therefore, expect that the highest rates of fat synthesis and fat storage would occur in airborne animals, since birds and flying insects have the greatest problem of working against gravity. However, all mobile animals living on the terrestrial parts of the planet have high rates of fat synthesis and fat storage, because this is the only way they can carry a large depot of calories and survive episodes when calories are not available from the environment.

A second reason why fat is extremely important to survival is that fat cells contain far more energy per gram than is contained in glycogen stores. The data (Fig. 1-2), derived decades ago by Dr. Wallace Fenn, show fat and carbohydrate as stored in tissue. At the right, is shown what happens to a cell when it increases its carbohydrate content. As is well known, carbohydrate is stored in the form of glycogen. Dr. Fenn showed that for every gram of glycogen that is stored, about 1.5-2 g of water are

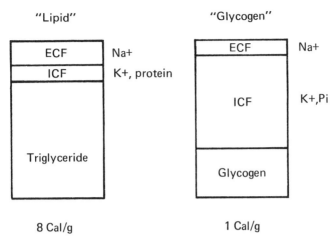

Fig 1-2. Composition of tissues storing lipid and glycogen. In adipose tissue stores (*left*), triglyceride is the predominant storage form and such tissues contain approximately 8 kCal/g. For glycogen-containing tissues (*right*), the energy stored is dissolved in the intracellular fluid and the energy content is thus much reduced approximately 1 kCal/g.

required. Thus, as the cell expands its glycogen content, water has to be imbibed and isotonicity has to be maintained. Electrolytes, including potassium, phosphate, and magnesium, also move into the cell. Therefore, when a cell expands its carbohydrate depot, it accumulates only 1 or 1.5 Cal/g of total tissue. This is a poor way to store energy if you have to carry it around with you!

Fig. 1-3. Lipogenesis from glucose. The process of converting glucose into fatty acids converts energy from an inefficiently stored molecule (glucose) into fatty acids, which can be stored with higher caloric density.

$$C_6H_{12}O_6 \longrightarrow \begin{array}{c} -CH_2\,CH_2- \\ \\ -CH_2\ CH_2- \end{array} \quad +2\,CO_2\ +2\,H_2O$$

Glucose   Added to fatty acid

The other bar (Fig. 1-2) shows that when a cell increases its lipid content, most of what is stored is triglyceride or lipid itself. There is a little increase in intracellular fluid, and a little increase in extracellular fluid as the cells enlarge, but the greatest proportion of the expansion is the lipid. When lipid expands, it yields close to the theoretical 9.4 Cal/g. The process of lipogenesis (Fig. 1-3) or fat synthesis converts the energy from carbohydrates into fat. When we eat carbohydrate and make fat, we're turning a poor economy-type fuel into a good economy-type fuel.

Each and every one of us has, for practical purposes, an optimally expanded total-body nitrogen pool. Even if we were to eat another pound or two of steak in one day, we would produce only a small increase in body nitrogen and the next day we would probably get rid of it. In other words, we are ideally expanded in terms of protein for the average amount of exercise we get. Any extra protein that is taken in will be converted into fat and stored as such.

Less well known is the fact that most of us (except when we wake up in the morning) have optimally expanded our total-body glycogen stores to about 6% in liver and 1% in muscle. Extra calories that are taken in, in the form of carbohydrate, are converted into fat for storage.

The problem is that once we have crossed the synthetic pathway from carbohydrate and amino acids to fatty acid, there is a point of no return (Fig. 1-4). Mammals are totally unable to convert fat back into carbohydrate or into amino acids. Once the fat has been synthesized and stored, the only thing that can happen to it is oxidization to CO_2 and water.

Recent data from liver biopsies have emphasized how relatively minimal are the glycogen stores in a normal man. In the normal liver, there is about 5-10% glycogen after eating. Following an overnight fast, liver glycogen content decreases markedly and for more prolonged fasts plasma glucose is maintained by gluconeogenesis rather than from glycogenolysis. The stores of carbohydrate in the liver are approximately 50-75 g, and is relatively small compared to the total daily caloric flux of 2000-3000 Cal. This is why I emphasize that all of us have glycogen stores which are nearly fully expanded and excess carbohydrate calories are formed into fat instead. In other words, adipose tissue is the caloric buffer that had to defend us against energy needs.

Conversely, if the diet be hypocaloric, providing there is a minimal amount of nitrogen, then the caloric deficit will be almost entirely met by

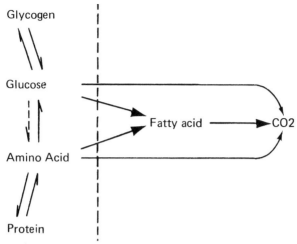

Fig. 1-4. Conversion of amino acids and glucose to fatty acids. The vertical dash line represents the irreversible reaction involved in conversion of carbons from glucose and amino acids into fatty acids. Although fatty acids can be oxidized to carbon dioxide in water, their carbons cannot be used for net synthesis of glucose or amino acids.

fat catabolism. A schematic presentation of blood glucose concentration through a 24-hour period of time is plotted in Figure 1-5. The serum insulin always responds to changes in the circulating fuel mixture. The important part of this figure is at the top and shows that after eating, we deposit fuel in our peripheral depots. Likewise, when we are not eating, we are mobilizing the fuels for bodily needs. The total area above and the total area below in all of us is just about equal from day to day. If a few extra calories are creeping in, the area above will be larger and we will gain weight. Conversely, if we are restricting food, the area below will be larger, and we will lose weight. In other words, the expansion or contraction of lipid in adipose tissue depends upon whether our state is relatively hypercaloric or hypocaloric. It appears that insulin directs these effects but does not initiate them. The amount of fuel that enters the body is the initiating event. In other words, insulin is the regulator responding to the drive generated by fuel ingestion.

Now let us focus on the physiology of insulin and its effects on the fat-cell membrane as they relate to the pathophysiology of obesity. In the past 3 years, several investigators have shown very clearly that insulin

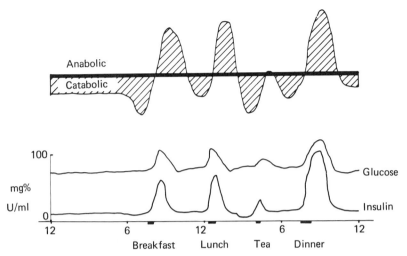

Fig. 1-5. Glucose and insulin throughout the 24 hours. Following each meal there is a rise in glucose and insulin. These periods correspond with the anabolic portion at the top of the figure. In between these anabolic periods are the catabolic phases in which stored energy is released and oxidized.

Fig. 1-6. Schematic representation of action of insulin at the cell wall. A hypothesized second messenger is formed that is responsible for the enzyme effects and either directly or indirectly responsible for the insulin effects on cell-wall permeability.

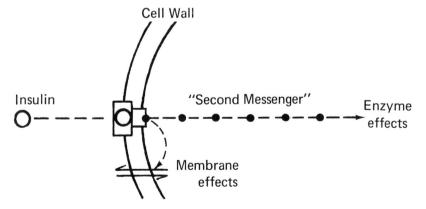

works on the cell membrane. Figure 1-6 is a simple graphic scheme to show a hypothetical cell wall and the effects of insulin. Insulin circulates in the extracellular fluids, and when it comes to a responsive cell, it binds to a specific receptor on the cell membrane. This receptor can identify insulin. The interaction of insulin and the receptor initiates some metabolic event, which then initiates several other events. One of these is that the membrane elsewhere in the cell changes its characteristics to facilitate the entry of glucose so it can be metabolized.

Without insulin, glucose will not enter these tissues. Adipose tissue needs insulin to let glucose in. Insulin also "tells" the previously stored fat inside the fat cell to stay there, and not to be broken down and released. In other words, insulin causes the lipolytic mechanism of the fat cell to slow up. These effects of insulin on the cell membrane appear to be due to some second messenger that insulin sets up inside the cell. We do not yet know what this signal is. Cyclic AMP is a second messenger for many tissues, but as far as insulin is concerned, cyclic AMP, either increased or decreased, is probably not the only signal.

Insulin also initiates different patterns of enzymes within the cell. One of the pathologic sequelae in persons who are overweight is that it takes more insulin to do whatever insulin does to the fat cell. Cuatrecasas even characterized the number of insulin molecules needed to bind to the normal and abnormal fat cell (2). The null point illustrated in Figure 1-7, where anabolic events lie on one side and catabolic events on the other, is that concentration of insulin which is present in physiologic fluids. This concentration is approximately the same as that which half-saturates the binding sites on the cell membrane—*i.e.,* the "Km" to the biochemist. Insulin appears to bind to the receptive cells, and the concentration of insulin required to bind to half the sites on these responsive cells is the physiologic concentration of insulin that appears in normal people but not in the overweight population. Overweight people need much more insulin.

Now what does this all mean? It means, in the first place, that fat is the caloric buffer to the environment. It also means that insulin is the primary controller of the fat cell, telling the fat cell, when adequate fuel is present, to take up the fuel and to store it therein. Not only does glucose go into fat, but fat which we eat also goes into fat in excess, as long as there is enough insulin around. In certain situations, particularly in obesity, fat cells need more insulin for each one of the metabolic events it controls. Moreover, other body tissues in the obese individual also need more

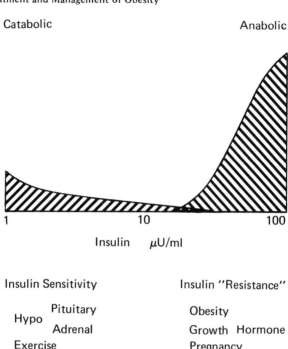

Fig. 1-7. Catabolic and anabolic effects of insulin. When high concentrations of insulin are required for anabolic effects, insulin resistance is present. In certain states, insulin sensitivity increases and low concentrations of plasma insulin are present.

insulin. The muscle cells appear to need more insulin, so the metabolic sequelae of an expanded fat store that occur with obesity are not limited to the fat cell but take place in many other tissues as well.

METABOLIC ASPECTS OF STARVATION

The amount of glucose stored in liver as glycogen is only enough to support fasting for several hours, as mentioned before. Therefore, the bulk of the glucose that is made after an overnight fast must be made *de novo* in the liver from amino acids coming from muscle. This is why protein breakdown occurs and nitrogen loss develops during total starvation. The amino acids from muscle are released into the blood and are taken up by the liver to make glucose to supply the needs of the brain. Other tissues in the body, such as the red cells, the kidney medulla, white cells, peripheral nerves, etc., also use glucose as their primary fuel. These tissues, however, do not oxidize the glucose all the way to CO_2 as the brain does, but instead metabolize the glucose to lactic acid. This acid reenters the bloodstream and is carried back to the liver, where it is remade into glucose. This cycle of glucose to lactic acid and back to glucose was described by Dr. Carl Cori some 50 years ago and is called the Cori cycle (3). What happens to the rest of the carcass during starvation? What keeps the muscles, heart, spleen, kidney cortex, and all the other tissues going when we are not eating? The major fuel for these tissues is fatty acids which come from adipose tissue. Some of the fatty acids get into these tissues indirectly by going through the liver and being made into keto acids.

The metabolic requirements during fasting are diagrammed in Figure 1-8. A normal may lying down for a 24-hour period will utilize about 1800 Cal. During this time, he will need about 75 g protein, which is equivalent

Fig. 1-8. Metabolic requirements during fasting (24 hours basal: 1800 Cal). *At left,* origin of fuel from muscle and adipose tissues and its approximate contribution. *At right,* fuel consumption by nerve, blood cells, and heart, kidney, and muscle are shown.

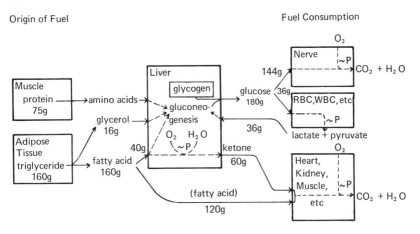

to 300 g lean muscle. But this is only about one-fifth of his total caloric expenditure. The rest of the calories he is burning come from fat in the adipose tissue. This number of calories represents about 160 g triglyceride or one-third of a pound of fat. If a person eats 3000 Cal and burns 2000 Cal, the 1000-Cal difference will be made into fat and stored. Conversely, as he burns 1000 Cal more than he consumes a day, the deficit will be made up by oxidation of fat. It should be reemphasized, however, that muscle loss accounts for about two-thirds of a pound of weight loss, and fat, for only about one-third of a pound in a man fasted for a single 24-hour period.

The question is: How does the muscle know that the brain needs a certain amount of sugar to be made by the liver? What is the feedback process that controls this entire scheme? There is an old observation that if one gives a normal, fasting person a small amount of carbohydrate by mouth or by vein, two major events will occur: (1) The mobilization of muscle protein will be markedly diminished; (2) the liver will no longer make glucose, because the small amount of sugar taken by mouth or by vein satisfies the brain's needs.

If we give our hypothetical fasting man a liter of 10% dextrose and water (this amount providing the glucose needed by his brain), we will spare the need for his liver to make glucose. The liver also will not make keto acids, and the mobilization of muscle nitrogen will also be spared. Instead of the 75 g protein per day that this man would mobilize were he not getting his glucose and water, he will mobilize only about 15 g protein.

Now, how does the muscle know how to hold on to its nitrogen when a little bit of glucose is infused? It is probably by way of insulin. Glucose will increase insulin release and this will tell the muscle to slow the breakdown of protein.

As the glucose level in the blood falls a little bit (Fig. 1-9), the thermostat—the pancreatic beta cells—will put out a little less insulin, and the muscle and the fat cells are thereby instructed to put a little more fatty acid and more amino acid into the blood. The liver will then make a little more sugar. The sugar level will increase, and the feedback cycle continues to maintain glucose within normal levels.

In short-term starvation, 75 g protein is used each day. If we continued to use muscle at this rate, we would not survive for more than a few weeks because we would have lost so much of our muscle. But, somehow, when starvation persists beyond several days, man uses less and less of his muscle nitrogen.

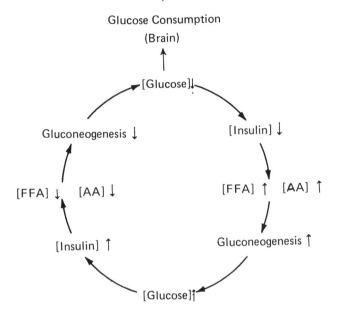

FFA = Free fatty acid
AA = Amino acid

Fig. 1-9. Schematic representation of control of blood glucose. Glucose utilization by the brain decreases plasma glucose, which leads to a drop in insulin, a rise in free fatty acids, and release of amino acids from their stored depots. This in turn stimulates glucogenesis and restores the glucose concentration to normal. The rise in insulin shuts off release of amino acids and fatty acids and diminishes glucogenesis, thus leading to precise control of blood glucose.

Monitoring of urine nitrogen excretion during a 5-week fast in an overweight patient, shows that each day during the fast, the nitrogen level in the urine gets lower and lower (Fig. 1-10). That is, the subject is becoming more and more efficient in holding onto his muscle nitrogen. Initially, he was losing about 75 g protein or 12 g nitrogen a day. This gradually decreased to about 20 g protein. It would fall a little more slowly if the patient were to continue the fast for 3 or 4 months. How can this be explained? Apparently other substrates, mainly keto acids, appear in the blood and are able to displace the need of the brain to utilize glucose. The human produces three so-called "ketone bodies." Acetone is

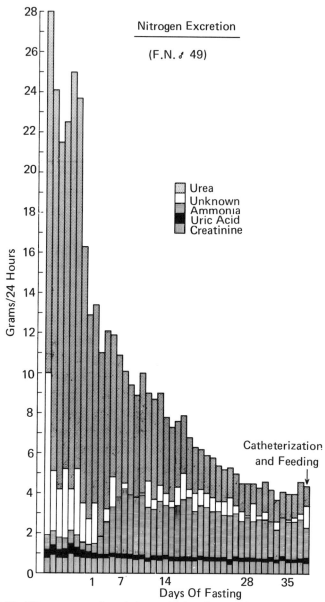

Fig. 1-10. Nitrogen excretion during a 39-day fast. During this time span, the quantity of urea excreted diminishes to small levels and the quantity of ammonia rises. With prolonged fasting, mechanisms for conserving nitrogen come in to play.

really a curiosity because it usually appears only in very low concentrations. It imparts a characteristic odor to the breath when it is in high concentration in the circulation. Acetone is also a metabolic dead end. The other two ketone bodies, beta-hydroxybutyrate and acetoacetate, are metabolically active.

The plasma level of ketones in prolonged starvation is of a higher concentration on a mole basis than is the concentration of glucose. In fasting, the blood is richer in ketone calories than in glucose calories. The important point is that the ketones plateau at about 6 or 7 mEq (normal bicarbonate of 25-27). It is a mild, balanced, and regulated acidosis but, so far as we can tell, poses no threat to the patient because it does not become excessive.

With prolonged starvation, the brain begins to use ketones (Fig. 1-11) and somehow signals the muscles, possibly through insulin, that now the brain can use ketones, amino acids are no longer necessary for gluconeogenesis. With the lower rate of nitrogen mobilization, the stores of body nitrogen in an average person will provide about 4 months of

Fig. 1-11. Metabolic fuels for the brain during prolonged starvation. Under normal circumstances (*at left*), glucose supplies essentially 100% of the fuel requirements for brain metabolism. After adaptation to "starvation," the brain decreases its requirements for glucose and adapts to utilizing betahydroxybutyrate, acetoacetate, and the carbons from α-amino nitrogen.

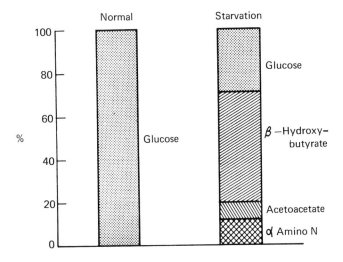

Origin of Fuel   Fuel Consumption

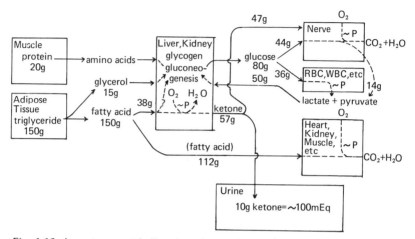

Fig. 1-12. Long-term metabolic adaptation to fasting (24 hours basal: 1500 Cal). After 5–6 weeks of fasting, the source of metabolic fuels is altered from that observed with short-term fasting (Fig. 1-8). The quantity of amino acids provided by muscle declines from 75 to 20 g, while the quantity of triglyceride hydrolized remains nearly the same. The utilization of glucose by nerve and brain declines from 144 to 44 g, and the difference is made up by the oxidation of ketone bodies produced in the liver from fatty acids.

gluconeogenesis at this remarkably reduced rate that begins after a week or two of total starvation (Fig. 1-12).

REFERENCES

1. Cahill GF Jr: Physiology of insulin in man. Diabetes 20:785-799, 1971.
2. Cori CF: Physiol Rev 11:143-000, 1931.
3. Cuatrecasas P: Insulin-receptor interactions in adipose tissue cells: direct measurement and properties. Proc Natl Acad Sci (USA) 68:1264-1268. 1971.

Cellularity of Adipose Tissue

2

LESTER B. SALANS

Obesity is a disorder in which there is an abnormal enlargement of the adipose tissue mass. Associated with this excessive accumulation of body fat are abnormalities of carbohydrate (25) and lipid metabolism (24), and of insulin secretion (1, 20) and its action (11). During the past several years a considerable amount of investigative attention has been directed toward the nature of the adipose tissue in obesity and the role of the adipose cell in the genesis and perpetuation of the obese state and its associated metabolic abnormalities. This discussion will review some of the recent investigations into the morphologic and metabolic character of the adipose tissue in obesity.

Enlargement of the adipose tissue in the obese individual represents an excessive accumulation of calories. These excess calories are stored in adipose cells in the form of triglyceride. Anatomically this may be accomplished either by storing the increased amount of triglyceride in preexisting adipose cells (increased cell size), or by the formation of new adipocytes (increased cell number). The development of reliable methods for determining the triglyceride content of fat cells (cell size) in isolated pieces of adipose tissue and for estimating the total number of adipocytes in the body (3, 15, 34) has enabled a study of the cellular character of the adipose tissue during normal growth in the nonobese state and during its abnormal growth in obesity.

Such studies indicate that adipose tissue normally grows by an orderly process of increasing adipose cell number and size (16). Early in life, cellular multiplication is the predominant factor responsible for the growth of the adipose tissue, but later, cell number becomes fixed, and thereafter, the adipose tissue expands, or shrinks, almost exclusively by changes in fat cell size (30). The exact age at which final cell number is reached, and subsequently remains constant, is not yet known, but it appears that this state is reached at around 20 years of age, or perhaps earlier (27). Estimates of total adipose cell number in nonobese adults range from 20 to 46×10^9 (27). Adipose cell size in these nonobese patients may vary considerably from one fat depot to another—from 0.20 to 0.70 μg lipid per cell, depending upon the depot examined.

In obesity there is a derangement of this orderly process of growth in the adipose tissue; alterations may occur in adipose cell size, cell number, or both. Two abnormal cellular patterns have been described in the expanded adipose depot of obese patients.

The first type is characterized by hypercellularity of the adipose tissue (2, 16, 27). These obese persons may have mild (58×10^9) to marked (155×10^9) increases in total adipose cell number, the latter usually occurring in the most massively obese. Adipose cell size in this type of obesity may be either normal or enlarged. This type of obesity begins, almost without exception, early in life; in general, the earlier the age of onset, the greater the hypercellularity of the adipose depot and the more severe the obesity. There appear to be two periods in early life when hypercellularity is most likely to develop: very early, within the first few years, and later, at or around the time of puberty. Patients with onset of obesity within the first few years of life have the greatest increase in cell number and the most nearly normal cell size, while those with onset at puberty have smaller degrees of hypercellularity, and larger fat cells.

A second pattern of obesity is characterized by the presence of enlarged, but normal numbers of adipose cells in the expanded adipose depot (2, 3, 16, 27, 30). This type of obesity begins in adult life, and is usually mild to moderate in severity. The exact age at which hypercellularity can no longer occur and at which the adipose depot expands through the storage of the excess calories in preexisting adipocytes is not known with certainty, but except in rare instances, this probably occurs before the age of 20 years.

The possible significance of these observations becomes apparent when one considers the additional observation that weight reduction in all obese patients, regardless of age of onset or degree and duration of obesity, has so far been shown to be achieved by virtue of a change in adipose cell size only; cell number remains constant even in the face of massive degrees of weight loss (16, 30). Thus, it appears that the hypercellularity of the adipose depot of the patient with early-onset, massive obesity is irreversible. This anatomic phenomenon is paralleled by the well-known and frustrating clinical observation that weight reduction in the lifelong, severely obese patient is almost inevitably followed by regain of weight and restoration of the original state of adiposity. Indeed, the inadequacy of current dietary approaches to the problem of obesity may be due to their inability to effect any permanent change in adipose tissue cellularity in adult life.

This pessimistic view must be tempered by the fact that no determination has yet been made of cell number in this type of obese patient after prolonged periods at reduced weight. It remains possible that under such circumstances cell number may decrease. However, the currently available studies are in general agreement that adipose hypercellularity, once established, is permanent. In view of this, and of the apparent age-related nature of this phenomenon, considerable attention has been focused on early life and on the factors that influence adipose cellular division and the early growth of the adipose tissue. Elucidation of these factors might permit more successful therapeutic approaches toward modification of adipose cellularity and, thus, prevention or control of obesity. Of particular interest in this respect is the observation by Knittle and Hirsch (23) that early nutritional experiences can permanently modify adipose cell number in the rat. These investigators reported that manipulation of total caloric intake during neonatal life in the rat induced changes in adipose cell number that persisted throughout the life of the animal and were associated with a permanent alteration in body weight and adiposity. Similar nutritional influences may operate early in the life of man; in particular, overeating at this stage of life may induce hypercellularity of the adipose tissue and, as a consequence, obesity. Thus, the importance of avoiding overnutrition in early life has been stressed.

Obviously, other endocrine, nutritional, and genetic determinants of adipose cell number must be examined. Considerable speculation has centered on the effect of insulin on the growth of the adipose tissue. The anabolic effects of this hormone are well known, particularly with respect to triglyceride metabolism, and an excessive amount of insulin is frequently observed in the blood of obese patients. An examination of the influence of insulin on the growth of rat adipose tissue, however, indicates that this hormone stimulates the growth of this tissue solely by increasing fat cell size (32, 36). Even when insulin is administered in the neonatal period, no increases in adipose cell number are observed. The effects of this and other hormones during intrauterine life, as well as the influences of maternal and fetal nutrition, on the growth of the adipose tissue must also be examined. Genetic factors have also been shown to influence the final morphology of the adipose tissue in a variety of experimental animals, the nature of the effect depending upon the time in life at which they act (18, 19). It might be of particular interest, and of some therapeutic benefit, to determine whether the factors operating to increase cell number during the first few years of life differ from those producing hypercellularity at puberty.

The mechanism by which adipose hypercellularity might act to perpetuate the obese state is unknown. One possibility is that an increased number of adipose cell number signals the hypothalmus, or higher feeding centers in the brain, to stimulate increased food intake. Kennedy (21) has postulated a lipostatic theory for the regulation of food intake, in which the feeding centers control, and in turn are regulated by, the total amount of fat in the body. It is possible that this feedback between the feeding centers of the central nervous system and the body fat is somehow mediated through adipose cell number. Thus, the presence of adipose hypercellularity, and its persistence even after weight reduction, may be the source of a permanent stimulus for excessive food intake and for restoration of the enlarged adipose mass. Clearly, this area requires further investigation.

These morphologic data, then, permit a new classification of obesity into juvenile and adult onset, and may provide the basis for a better understanding of and a more successful therapeutic approach to the problem. In addition, knowledge of the cellular character of the adipose tissue may also provide some insight into the metabolic consequences of obesity.

The concept that the disordered metabolic state of the obese patient is somehow related to the adipose tissue is based on the observation that glucose intolerance, hyperglycemia, hyperinsulinemia, and hypertriglyceridemia are frequently present when the patient is obese, but disappear with weight loss (1, 20, 24, 25, 31). Moreover, the findings that normal glucose tolerance in the obese is maintained only in the face of very high concentrations of plasma insulin and that this, too, is completely reversible by weight reduction suggest that these metabolic abnormalities may be related to the nature of the adipose tissue itself. Since adipose cellular enlargement is common to both types of obesity and adipose cell size is the only morphologic characteristic that is reversible with weight reduction, particular interest has centered on the possible role of fat cell size in this apparent relationship between the adipose tissue and the general metabolic abnormalities of the obese.

The metabolic activity of the adipose tissue of a large number of nonobese and obese patients has been examined as a function of adipose cell size, and these *in vitro* relationships have been correlated with simultaneous *in vivo* measurements, made in the plasma and in forearm tissue, of glucose, lipid, and insulin metabolism. The influence of diet on these relationships has also been examined.

A proper evaluation and interpretation of these relationships requires that the state of becoming obese must be distinguished from the state of being obese (28). During the process of becoming obese, the lipogenic function of the adipose cell is, quite obviously, hyperactive; at the same time its lipolytic activity is diminished (6). This appears to be the result of increased substrate delivery to the cell—*i.e.*, excessive ingestion and absorption of calories—rather than the result of some intrinsic cellular abnormality. Glucose appears to be a good substrate for lipogenesis in the adipose cell at this time (4). During this phase of active weight gain or of becoming obese, the adipose cell is hypersensitive to insulin—exquisitely so, perhaps (6, 28). All of these changes are even more marked when the individual is ingesting a diet high in carbohydrate (29).

As the cell enlarges with triglyceride, and once a steady state of obesity has been reached, certain adaptive changes occur. The ability of insulin to influence several aspects of glucose metabolism by enlarged adipose cells is diminished when compared to small cells. The lipolytic activity of the enlarged cell is enhanced, as indicated by an increased rate of release of glycerol and free fatty acid from the cell (6, 22, 33) and an accumulation of intracellular free fatty acid (6). At the same time, the enlarged adipocyte of the obese individual shows an increased capacity for esterification of fatty acid, as measured by an increased rate of glucose incorporation into triglyceride glycerol (12, 22, 28, 33). Thus, a paradoxical situation exists in which the enlarged cell continues to store triglyceride at an increased rate—*i.e.*, it remains large—in the face of adaptive changes, such as insulin resistance and enhanced lipolysis, which are operating to make the cell smaller by preventing further storage of calories as triglyceride. Net triglyceride turnover in the enlarged cell is, therefore, proceeding at an increased rate, compared to the small cell, and maintenance of the "fat-stuffed" state must reflect a higher equilibrium between the lipogenic and lipolytic function of the cell.

The most likely mechanism for the maintenance of cell size in the face of insulin resistance and enhanced lipolysis that the obese patient continues to ingest large amounts of food, and that the adaptive changes at the cellular level are overcome by the continued delivery of excessive lipogenic substrate to the cell. In contrast to the situation observed during the process of becoming obese, where glucose is a good source for the increased lipogenesis in the adipose cell, the enlarged adipocyte of the individual who has achieved a steady state of obesity appears to reside in the fat, has only a very limited capacity for glucose lipogenesis. This is consistent with the observation that, in man in a steady state of weight, the adipose tissue apparently accounts for only a very small fraction of the total glucose utilized by the body (26). Thus, speculation centers on fatty acid, and more specifically, lipoprotein, as the substrate for the enhanced lipogenesis occurring in the enlarged adipose cell.

These observations establish the alterations in glucose and lipid metabolism and the impairment of insulin action in the enlarged adipose cell of the obese individual. All of these cellular abnormalities are reversible with weight loss and reduction of cell size. Furthermore, the *in vitro* metabolism of the adipose tissue and its relationship to cell size have been shown to be closely associated with the general state of glucose, lipid, and insulin metabolism, as measured, *in vivo* in the plasma (17, 29, 31, 33). Glucose intolerance, hypertriglyceridemia, and hyperinsulinemia are present in the obese state, when the metabolic function of the enlarged adipose cell is altered, and these general metabolic abnormalities disappear with weight loss and restoration of normal metabolism in the smaller adipose cell. Thus, it has been tempting to postulate that the general state of disordered metabolism in the obese patient can somehow be explained by a resistance to glucose metabolism in the adipose cell.

Although this is an attractive hypothesis, a number of studies indicate that the explanation requires more than just a consideration of adipose tissue metabolism and the influence of fat-cell size. As discussed previously, apparently only a small fraction of the total glucose metabolism by the human body can be accounted for by the adipose tissue when a state of constant body weight exists. The evidence for this assertion is, however, based on studies conducted in the fasted state; it remains possible that glucose utilization by the adipose tissue may be significant in man during the fast state. An impairment of glucose metabolism by the adipose tissue of the obese is, however, unlikely to cause hyperglycemia or glucose intolerance by itself. It has been of considerable interest then to find that the adipose tissue is not the only tissue in the obese to undergo alterations in its metabolism. The stimulation of glucose uptake by insulin and the inhibition of amino acid release from skeletal muscle of obese patients by this hormone is also impaired (9, 17, 26). Insulin resistance of skeletal muscle in obesity is reversed by weight reduction concomitant with the reversion to normal that occurs in the adipose tissue. More recent studies indicate the liver of the obese individual may also be resistant to insulin.

These observations indicate a generalized impairment of insulin action in the tissues of the obese individual. Which of these tissues, if any, is primarily responsible for the altered state of glucose and lipid metabolism and for hyperinsulinemia and insulin resistance in the obese state, or how they interact to produce these abnormalities, is unknown. These findings also imply the existence of a feedback mechanism operating between the "insulin-resistant" peripheral tissue and the beta cell of the pancreas. The nature of this feedback has been the source of recent speculation (10, 37). It should be pointed out that hyperinsulinemia in the obese individual often occurs in the presence of normal concentration of blood glucose. Thus, it is unlikely that glucose is the primary signal to the pancreas for excessive insulin secretion. Some other mediator may be operative and may yet be a function of the adipose cell size. The enlarged adipose cell may, for example, secrete a substance which acts directly on the beta cell to increase its secretion of insulin, or which acts indirectly by altering the muscle and/or the liver, thereby influencing the beta cell through these tissues.

Although these alterations in tissue metabolism provide an excellent base upon which to speculate, the contribution of the dietary intake of the obese individual to the disordered metabolic state should not be overlooked. Increased ingestion and turnover of calories is, in itself, associated with an increased requirement for insulin and a change in the general metabolic state. Several recent studies indicate that the character of adipose tissue metabolism, as well as the state of glucose tolerance and the concentration of triglyceride and insulin in the plasma, are influenced by the amount and the nature of the diet being ingested (4, 5, 7, 14, 17, 28, 29, 33). As discussed previously, the metabolic activity of the adipose tissue during the phase of active weight gain differs significantly from that observed once a steady state of obesity has been reached. These observations indicate that the metabolic alterations observed in obesity reflect the response of the individual not only to the presence of excessive adiposity, but also to the nature of the diet. Preliminary attempts to dissociate the effect of diet from that of adiposity indicate that both factors interact to produce the altered metabolic state of the obese (17).

It is obvious from the foregoing discussion that additional studies are required to unravel the complexities of human obesity and the role of the fat cell in the genesis and perpetuation of the obese state and its associated metabolic abnormalities. It should also be obvious from this discussion that to obtain meaningful information about these relationships, the type of obesity must be defined in cellular terms, and the studies must be conducted under well-defined and carefully controlled conditions of body weight and dietary intake.

REFERENCES

1. Bagdade JD, Bierman EL, Porte D: The significance of basal insulin levels in the evaluation of the insulin response to glucose in diabetic and nondiabetic subjects. J Clin Invest 46:1549-1557, 1967

2. Björntorp P, Sjöström L: Number and size of adipose tissue fat cells in relation to metabolism in human obesity. Metabolism 20:703-713, 1971

3. Bray GA: Measurement of subcutaneous fat cells from obese patients. Ann Intern Med 73:565-569, 1970

4. Bray GA: Lipogenesis in human adipose tissue: some effects of nibbling and gorging. J Clin Invest 51:537-548, 1972

5. Brunzell JD, Lerner RL, Hazzard WR, Porte D Jr, Bierman EL: Improved glucose tolerance with high carbohydrate feeding in mild diabetes. N Eng J Med 284:521-524, 1971

6. Cushman SW, Salans LB: Cell associated fatty acids: a role in the mediation of cell size effects on adipose cell function. Clin Res XXI:620, 1973

7. Farquhar JW, Frank A, Gross RC, Reaven GM: Glucose, insulin, and triglyceride responses to high and low carbohydrate diets in man. J Clin Invest 45:1648-1656, 1966

8. Felig PE, Wahren J, Hendler R, Brundin T: Obesity: Evidence of heptatic resistance to insulin. Clin Res 21:623, 1973

9. Felig P, Horton ES, Runge CF, Sims EAH: Experimental obesity in man: hyperaminoacidemia and diminished effectiveness of insulin in regulative peripheral amino acid release. 53rd Meeting, Endocrine Society, 1971

10. Felig P, Marliss E, Cahil GF Jr: Plasma amino acid levels and insulin secretion in obesity. N Eng J Med 281:811-816, 1969

11. Franckson JR, Malaise W, Arnould Y, Rasio E, Ooms HA, Balasse E, Conard V, Bastenie PA: Glucose kinetics in human obesity. Diabetologica 2:96-103, 1966

12. Goldrick RB, McLoughlin GM: Lipolysis and lipogenesis from glucose in human fat cells of different sizes: effects of insulin, epinephrine, and theophylline. J Clin Invest 49:1213-1233, 1970

13. Greenwood MRC, Johnson PR, Hirsch J: The effect of age on the size and metabolic activity of isolated adipose cells from C57B mice. Fed Proc 28:688, 1969

14. Grey N, Kipnis DM: Effect of diet composition on the hyper-insulinemia of obesity. N Eng J Med 285:827-831, 1971

15. Hirsch J, Gallian E: Methods for the determination of adipose cell size in man and animals. J Lipid Res 9:110-110, 1968

16. Hirsch J, Knittle JL: Cellularity of obese and nonobese human adipose tissue. Fed Proc 29:1516-1521, 1970

17. Horton E, Danforth E, Sims EAH, Salans LB: Correlation of forearm muscle and adipose tissue metabolism in obesity before and after weight loss. Clin Res 20:548, 1972

18. Johnson PR, Hirsch J: Cellularity of adipose depots in six strains of genetically obese mice. J Lipid Res 13:2-11, 1972

19. Johnson PR, Zucker LM, Cruce JAF, Hirsch J: Cellularity of adipose depots in the genetically obese Zucker rat. J Lipid Res 12:706-714, 1971

20. Karam JH, Grodsky GM, Forsham PH: Excessive insulin response to

glucose in obese subjects as measured by immunochemical assay. Diabetes 12:197-204, 1963

21. Kennedy GC: The role of depot fat in the hypothalamic control of food intake in the rat. Proc R Soc London [Biol] 140:578-592, 1953

22. Knittle JL, Fellner FG: Effect of weight reduction on *in vitro* adipose tissue lipolysis and cellularity in obese adolescents and adults. Diabetes 21:754-761, 1972

23. Knittle JL, Hirsch J: Effect of early nutrition on the development of rat epididymal fat pads: cellularity and metabolism. J Clin Invest 47:2091-2098, 1968

24. Lees RS, Wilson DE: The treatment of hyperlipidemia. N Eng J Med 284:186-195, 1971

25. Neuburgh LH: Control of the hyperglycemia of obese "diabetics" by weight reduction. Ann Intern Med 17:935-942, 1942

26. Rabinowitz D: Some endocrine and metabolic aspects of obesity. Ann Rev Med 21:241-254, 1970

27. Salans LB, Cushman SW, Weismann R: Studies of human adipose tissue: adipose cell size and number in nonobese and obese patients. J Clin Invest 52:929-941, 1973

28. Salans LB, Dougherty JW: The effect of insulin upon glucose metabolism by adipose cells of different size: influence of cell lipid and protein content, age, and nutritional state. J Clin Invest 50:1399-1410, 1971

29. Salans LB, Horton E, Sims EAH: Influence of fat cell size and dietary carbohydrate intake on adipose tissue insulin sensitivity in adult onset obesity. Clin Res 18:463, 1970

30. Salans LB, Horton ES, Sims EAH: Experimental obesity in man: cellular character of the adipose tissue. J Clin Invest 50:1005-1011, 1971

31. Salans LB, Knittle JL, Hirsch J: The role of adipose cell size and adipose tissue insulin sensitivity in the carbohydrate intolerance of human obesity. J Clin Invest 47:153-165, 1968

32. Salans LB, Zarnowski MJ, Segal R: Effect of insulin upon the cellular character of rat adipose tissue. J Lipid Res 13:616-623, 1972

33. Sims EAH, Danforth E Jr, Horton ES, Bray GA, Glennon JA, Salans LB: Endocrine and metabolic effects of experimental obesity in man. Rec Prog Horm Res 29:457-470, 1973

34. Sjöström L, Björntorp P, Vrana J: Microscopic fat cell size measurements on frozen-cut adipose tissue in comparison with automatic

determinations of osmium-fixed fat cells. J Lipid Res 12:521-530, 1971

35. Smith U: Effect of cell size on lipid synthesis by human adipose tissue *in vitro.* J Lipid Res 12:65-70, 1971

36. Vost A, Hollenberg CH: Effects of diabetes and insulin on DNA synthesis in rat adipose tissue. Endocrinology 87:606-610, 1970

37. Wise JK, Salans LB: Stimulation of insulin secretion by adipose tissue: effect of fat cell size. J Clin Invest 49:1032-1042, 1970

Studies in Human Hyperphagia

3

ETHAN A. H. SIMS

For the past 6 years the endocrine-metabolic group at University of Vermont College of Medicine has been engaged in an unusual occupation. In contrast to most workers in the field of obesity, we have been persuading lean people to gain weight. We have done this in the hope of increasing our understanding of the changes in spontaneous obesity and particularly its obscure relationship to diabetes. From radioimmunoassay studies it was clear that glucose tolerance and insulin, cortisol, and growth hormone response in human obesity differed from the findings in lean people. What was not clear was whether these changes were primary and perhaps important in causing the obesity or might be merely secondary to obesity and overeating. One logical way to attack this question was to enlist the interest of normal male volunteers with no family history of obesity or of diabetes and deliberately overfeed them so that the changes resulting from pure exogenous obesity could be studied.

My interest in this approach to the question of the metabolic changes in

Aided by grants from the United States Public Health Service: USPHS 5 R01 AM-10254 (Dr. Sims) and USPHS FR 00109 (Clinical Research Center).

obesity began in 1964 when I was working in Dr. Bernard Landau's laboratory at Western Reserve on the development of diabetes in Chinese hamsters. These animals develop diabetes that is similar to juvenile diabetes in man, but they never become obese. Many other strains of rodents which spontaneously develop hyperglycemia also become obese in spite of having large amounts of plasma insulin. These responses seem reasonable since the temporary accumulation of fat in anticipation of a period of famine is a natural and almost universal process. The woodchuck is a good example of this. He eats busily, gaining up to 50% above his basal weight during the late summer and fall and will lose it all by spring. Parenthetically, it is of interest in this species that during the period when the weight increases so strikingly the intake of food actually decreases even though activity is not grossly reduced. When we understand how this is brought about, we may know more about human obesity.

Four university students volunteered in the first attempt to gain but found that while they continued their normal curricular and extra-curricular activities they had difficulty in adding even 10% to their normal weight. This was the first finding which made us realize that obesity in young people may not be a simple behavioral problem of overeating.

When it became clear to us that, for normal young people, gaining weight would have to be a full-time job, we suggested a project of experimental weight gain to the warden of the Vermont State Prison. The warden believed that for the inmates to engage even in this somewhat unusual project might have some rehabilitative dividends and gave it his support. Accordingly we installed a dining-room, special kitchen facilities, and a recreation-TV room in the hospital area of the institution, and three custodial officers were enlisted to supervise the program.

Our studies to date have included the results on four groups of volunteers at the State Prison and two at the University. In all, 22 volunteers have achieved a gain in weight of 20% or more. Many of the data on these subjects have been reported elsewhere (11, 14-16). This report will emphasize certain aspects of the study which shed some light upon questions about spontaneously obese people.

WEIGHT GAIN BY DELIBERATE OVEREATING

Can a normally lean young person gain weight by deliberately overeating? The answer is a qualified Yes. Of those who do gain successfully, however, most have to work very hard at it. Some gain relatively easily, but only by dint of taking in a large number of calories. Figure 3-1 shows a young volunteer who doubled his adipose tissue mass and temporarily altered his body contours. This 50-kg man ingested up to 7000 Cal/day (Fig. 3-2). He required a large intake just to maintain the increased weight during the period of retesting. Most young volunteers can maintain their usual weight by eating an average of 1800 kCal/sq m body surface area, but it requires half again as many calories, or an average of 2700/sq m, for them to maintain the added 15-25% of body weight. Thus

Fig. 3-1. A member of the first group of volunteers, before and after increasing his weight 25% by overeating. Note doubling of body fat.

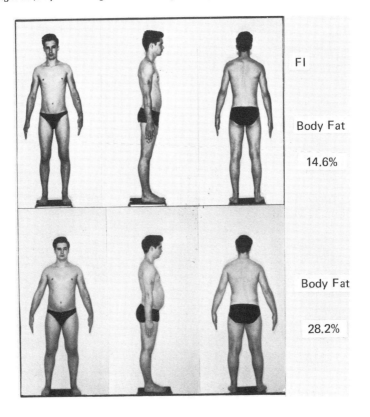

FI

Body Fat

14.6%

Body Fat

28.2%

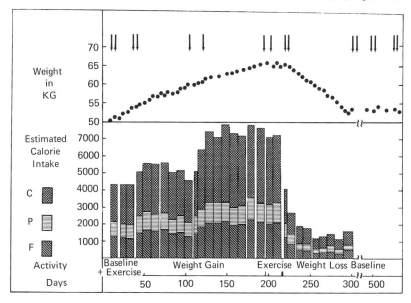

Fig. 3-2. Gain in weight in relation to caloric intake of the subject shown in Figure 3-1. Carbohydrate (*crosshatched*), protein (*horizontal shading*), and fat (*slant*) are shown in proportion to composition of diet by weight. Note large caloric intake required both to accomplish gain and maintenance of weight. (Sims EAH, Goldman RF, Gluck CM, Horton ES, Kelleher PC, Rowe DW: Experimental obesity in man. Trans Assoc Am Physicians 81:153-170, 1968)

3100 would maintain weight initially, whereas 5100 kCal are required after gaining weight.

This is reminiscent of the concept which was brought forth at the turn of the century in Germany under the name of "Luxuskonsumption." Neumann (10) performed a marathon experiment in which he varied his own intake of calories over a wide range and concluded that in the face of excessive caloric intake some type of metabolic wheel-spinning may take place in which some of the excess ingested calories are dissipated as heat rather than being used for mechanical work or for storage. There is conflicting evidence as to whether such a phenomenon in fact exists, and if so, as to where the extra calories go. In our studies it appears that there may be adaptive changes of this sort, particularly in some individuals taking a mixed diet, but we do not have completely balanced studies as yet. Similar deficits have been observed by Bray *et al.* (2) in four subjects. Various explanations for such deficits have been offered, but none have been validated. An increase in basal requirements for oxygen throughout the day in subjects given excess calories has been reported by Apfelbaum *et al.* (1). Moreover Miller, *et al.* (8) have suggested that the oxygen requirements for a given physical activity as well as those associated with the thermic effect of metabolizing a meal are increased during overfeeding. Bray *et al.* (2) have been unable to demonstrate any decreased efficiency of muscular contraction in four subjects who voluntarily took 4000 extra calories per day for a month. Dr. Haisman and Dr. Goldman at the Army Laboratories at Natick, Mass., (unpublished observations) have measured heat production and the response to meals and activity in one group of volunteers who gained weight in prison. At present only the basal studies have been completed. (4)

Whatever the mechanism, it is apparent that normal individuals may vary markedly in their ability to convert food into body mass. In Figure 3-3 are shown graphically the courses of two subjects whose dietary intake was accurately controlled for two periods of 3 weeks before and after gaining weight by increasing all elements of the diet. This was accomplished by employing uniform lots of TV dinners, suitably supplemented. Note that Volunteer P.T. (Fig. 3-3, *top*) gained readily while taking relatively few calories above his baseline requirement. Note also, that he still required a third more calories to maintain his weight. In contrast, the other subject (P.W.) ate a great deal, averaging 3400 Cal/day for a number of weeks, but gained relatively little, and was unable to add 20% to his body weight. Even 2700 Cal/sq m was inadequate to maintain what weight he did gain. In contrast to this, the usual severely obese patient requires only 1100-1300 kCal/sq m body surface area to maintain his weight, approximately half that of our modestly obese normal subject. Perhaps, however, a more valid comparison would be caloric requirements in terms of lean body mass, although it is difficult to arrive at a valid basis of comparison.

EFFECT OF OVEREATING ON FAT CELLS

Can one affect the number of adipose tissue cells by acute overeating? The answer is a qualified No. In our first two groups of volunteers the site of the adipose cells correlated closely with the increase in body fat,

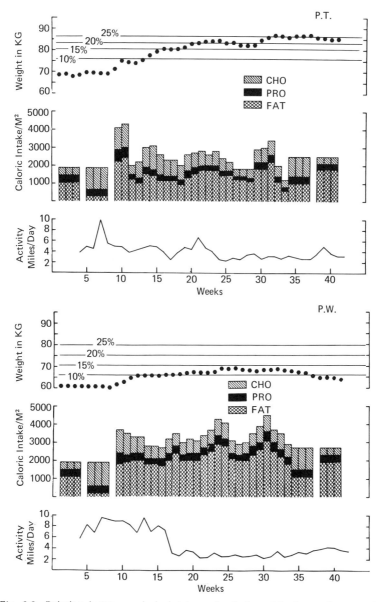

Fig. 3-3. Relation between caloric intake and gain in weight in a volunteer who gained readily (P.T.) contrasted with one who gained with difficulty and could not achieve his goal in spite of high caloric intake. *CHO* (*slant*), carbohydrate; *PRO* (*solid*), protein; and *FAT* (*crosshatch*), fat. Caloric intake is given per square meter of body surface area. The percent scale refers to gain above basal weight. Activity was crudely monitored by means of a pedometer. (Hormone and Metabolic Research.)

suggesting no change in number. In later groups Salans (13) estimated total cell number from measurements of adipose cell lipid content in three different areas of the body and, within limits of the technique, could demonstrate no change in the number of cells with gain in weight. But we cannot say that a more prolonged period of hyperphagia or of induced obesity might not have led to an increase in adipocyte number. Bray *et al.* (2) have presented evidence suggesting that young persons who develop obesity secondary to hypothalamic injury may increase their number of adipocytes. We should remember also that in spontaneous obesity the increase in cell number is not limited to adipose tissue. Naeye and Roode (9) have shown that in young obese accident victims there is both hyperplasia and hypertrophy of other body tissues as well.

DIFFERENCE BETWEEN EASY AND DIFFICULT WEIGHT GAIN

What determines whether a person gains weight easily or with difficulty? To obtain an approximate index of the difficulty in gaining weight we have used the number of calories per square meter of body surface area above the basal 1800 required to maintain weight, multiplied by the number of weeks required to add 20%. So far we have found no correlation of this index with the usual tests of thyroid function, change in cortisol metabolism, vanillylmandelic acid excretion as an index of catecholamine production, or the initial amount of lipid per adipose tissue cell. We do have a suggestion that the total number of adipose tissue cells with which one is endowed may be correlated with ability to gain weight (Fig. 3-4). On the other hand, when the number of cells for the three "hard-gaining" subjects, all of whom were somewhat small, is related to body surface area, there is a close correlation. We thus suspect that some unidentified factor simply may be related to smallness and that body cells other than fat cells may also share in the limitation in growth. Perhaps we shall know the answer when we understand the feedback mechanism which tells the central nervous system when an individual's normal is reached.

After having seen the difficulty that normal lean subjects have in attempting to gain weight, we are increasingly loath to disbelieve the patient who tells us, "Doctor, my neighbor eats like a horse and stays thin, while I really don't eat very much and gain. . . ." We may seriously add to the already great psychological burden of the obese patient if we regard his

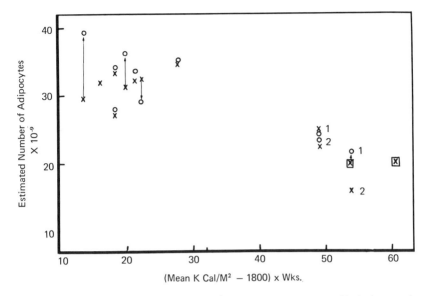

Fig. 3-4. Relation of ease of gain in weight (see text for explanation of index) to total number of body fat cells. X, initial estimate of cell number. O, final estimate of cell number. 1, initial study; 2, repeat study. The easily gaining subject P.T. of Figure 3-3 falls in the cluster in the left upper corner, while P.W., a hard gainer who made two attempts to gain, is third from the right. Adipocyte numbers are not corrected for body surface area or weight.

gaining weight purely as a matter of self-discipline, rather than a deep-seated and usually inherited problem of physiologic control.

EFFECTS OF OBESITY ON INSULIN

Does plasma insulin increase in experimental obesity as in spontaneous obesity? Does resistance to insulin also develop? In experimental obesity, as may be the case in spontaneous obesity, glucose tolerance was diminished, but like every other change in the overfed volunteers the values remained within the conventional range of normal (Fig. 3-5). There was an increase in basal insulin, and the secretion of insulin in response to glucose was also increased. The biological activity of the insulin suppressible by antiinsulin antibody was increased as well. Thus the ratio of insulin to glucose is increased, and we find the same paradox of decreased tolerance to glucose combined with increase in circulating insulin.

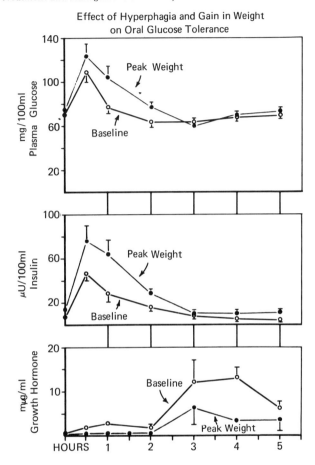

Fig. 3-5. Concentrations of glucose, insulin, and growth hormone in 11 subjects of the first two groups of volunteers prior to gain in weight (*open circles*) and following gain in weight (*closed circles*). Mean ± S.E.

Responses in plasma growth hormone are also blunted. The usual late rise in plasma growth hormone which follows an oral glucose load was reduced in the overfed volunteers as it is in spontaneous obesity. The spontaneous nocturnal rise was also blunted after weight gain. Although the production rate of cortisol is increased, the plasma concentration of cortisol is not increased in experimental obesity.

Consistent with the increase in plasma insulin and the insulin/glucose ratio, there is direct evidence of resistance to insulin in peripheral tissues. There is blunting of the sensitivity to insulin in adipose tissue obtained by biopsy from our volunteers with experimental obesity. However, since adipose tissue accounts for a relatively small fraction of glucose utilization, this alone could not explain the insulin resistance of experimental or spontaneous obesity. Some years ago Rabinowitz and Zierler (12) perfused the muscle of the forearm of normal and obese patients and found that obesity increased the basal glucose uptake and blunted the response to insulin. Similar perfusion studies by Horton in our overfed volunteers showed a similar blunting of the sensitivity of the muscle of the forearm to insulin after weight gain, but there was no change in basal glucose uptake (Fig. 3-6). Plasma amino acids were measured in plasma samples from the same perfusion studies (3). The data indicated that insulin had less effect on the release of branch-chain fatty acids from muscle after weight gain than before. Thus both muscle and fat cells become resistant to the action of insulin in experimental obesity. (14)

It should be emphasized that all we can conclude from these findings is that a modest degree of oversecretion of insulin and of insulin resistance may develop following overfeeding and gain in weight in normal subjects. However, these data do not rule out the possibility that in some of the syndromes of obesity, hypersecretion of insulin, or of some other hormone or circulating factor, could play a primary role in causing the disorder.

Also, we cannot say whether these changes are the result of some factor, as yet undefined, that is related to overnutrition and obesity, or whether, as Grey and Kipnis have suggested (5), the antecedent high intake of carbohydrate may not have led to hypersecretion of insulin, and whether in turn insulin resistance may have developed as a protection against the higher levels of insulin secretion. A number of studies carried out in our last two groups of volunteers suggest that both antecedent diet and the ratio of carbohydrate to fat may affect the response of adipose tissue and muscle to insulin (14). The studies are continuing. To test further the role of carbohydrate in producing the hyperinsulinemia, a group of volunteers in our Clinical Research Center gained weight while increasing dietary fat alone. The same degree of hyperinsulinism was found. Weight gain was surprisingly efficient and, in contrast to those in earlier groups, no added calories were required for maintenance (6).

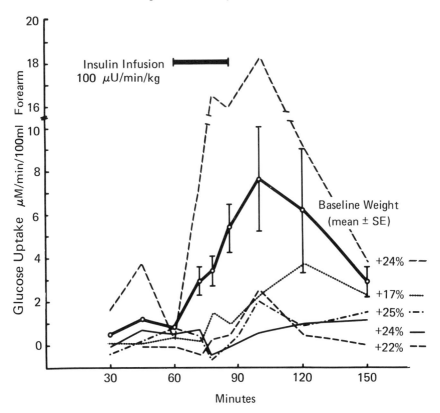

Fig. 3-6. Effect of arterial infusion of insulin on uptake of glucose by the deep venous bed of forearm before (*heavy solid line*) and after gain in weight. *At right*, the percent gain in weight by individual subjects. (Sims EAH, Danforth E Jr, Horton ES, Bray GA, Glennon JA, Salans LB: Endocrine and metabolic effects of experimental obesity in man. Recent Progr Horm Res)

EFFECTS OF WEIGHT GAIN ON ACTIVITY

Does overeating and gain in weight affect activity and initiative? This appears to be the case. Although there are no objective measurements, the men appeared to have less initiative and less spontaneous physical activity after gaining weight. In many instances their supervisors in the institution reported that the performance on work assignments was less satisfactory. Quite a few volunteers noted mild dyspnea on climbing a long flight of stairs to the third-floor dining area used for the study. Pulmonary function studies indicated a significant but moderate reduction in residual pulmonary volume.

APPETITE IN WEIGHT GAIN

What effect does gain in weight have upon appetite? A majority of the men taking a diet of 6,000-10,000 calories actually reported hunger either at the end of the afternoon or during the day, although anorexia was the usual reaction when a high-fat diet was consumed. This did not correlate with any chemical change, however. Serial measurements of glucose and insulin at hourly intervals throughout the day in the third group of volunteers indicated a gradual increase of the concentrations of glucose and insulin just prior to each meal. There was also a greater release of insulin associated with meals later in the day, but no hypoglycemia was found as a ready explanation of the increase in hunger. Familiarity with glucose tolerance tests led us to expect large fluctuations in glucose and insulin throughout the day. However, the excursions during a day in which normal meals were taken (Fig. 3-7) were relatively limited. The means of the insulin concentrations, initially and during the entire period, following each of the meals before, during, and after gain in weight were charted (Fig. 3-8). During the day there was a progressive increase in insulin secretion, which tended to be more marked following a gain in weight. The concentrations of insulin just before each meal, reflecting the changing basal insulin secretion (horizontal lines within the bars in Fig. 3-8) also increase progressively as the day goes on. These increases in baseline appear to account for the increase in the total insulin secretion. The basal insulin was increased at peak weight only during the early part of the day. This escalation of insulin secretion was not related to any increase in plasma cortisol, since this did not differ appreciably during the course of the day at base and at peak weight.

HYPERLIPIDEMIA AND OBESITY

Is hyperlipidemia associated with experimental obesity? In the first report on this group of studies we indicated that there was a decrease in plasma free fatty acids associated with overeating and experimental obesity. Further studies, however, have shown that the decrease in free fatty acids is associated with a high intake of carbohydrate. In the small

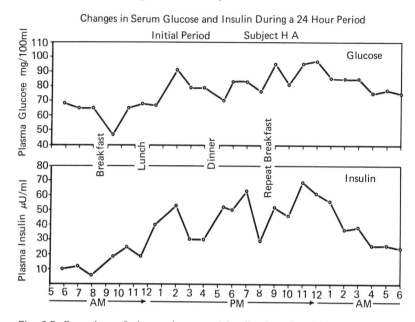

Fig. 3-7. Excursions of plasma glucose and insulin through a 24-hour period in a normal subject taking meals of usual composition throughout the day and repeating the breakfast at 8 P.M.

number of subjects studied, free fatty acids have not correlated with gain in weight when carbohydrate intake is controlled (14). When similar comparisons are made using controlled diets before and after gain in weight, serum *cholesterol* did not change with weight (14). The serum triglycerides were variably increased in association with increase in dietary carbohydrates, so that the changes with weight were not significant.

Thus an increase in weight alone is not necessarily correlated with any change in plasma lipids. As far as maintaining normal lipid concentrations is concerned, the important factors may be the level of intake of carbohydrate and other dietary factors, as well as the amount of increased physical activity in patients with spontaneous obesity.

CORTISOL METABOLISM

Is cortisol metabolism affected in experimental obesity? In spontaneous obesity the production rate of cortisol and the excretion of its metabolites

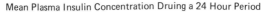
Mean Plasma Insulin Concentration Druing a 24 Hour Period

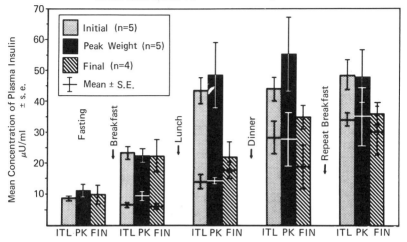

Fig. 3-8. Plasma insulin concentration during 24-hour period while fasting and during the period following three usual meals and a repeat breakfast at 8 P.M. before, during, and after gain in weight. Mean ± S.E. Means diagrammed within bars indicate concentration just prior to a particular meal. Note escalation of these baseline values throughout the day.

is increased, but only in proportion to the increase in body weight or surface area. The plasma concentration in uncomplicated obesity is either normal or reduced, suggesting an increase in its metabolic clearance. The studies in experimental obesity suggest that similar changes develop (11).

PERPETUATION OF ACQUIRED OBESITY

Are there factors which tend to perpetuate acquired obesity? There are quite a few such factors, including:

1. The diminished glucose uptake which would limit peripheral utilization in favor of fat deposition.
2. The increased plasma insulin which would promote the storage of carbohydrate and protein and would reduce lipolysis of adipocytes.
3. The reduced growth hormone response to various stimuli which also would tend to reduce lipolysis.
4. Enhanced appetite late in the day which would help to maintain intake

at the same time as reduced activity of evening and night hours would conserve fuels.

In earlier reports we emphasized that this series of changes could have survival value for a man or animal subjected to periodic famine. According to this line of reasoning, our volunteers should have tended to retain their weight, while in fact they did exactly the opposite. Essentially all of the subjects to date have lost weight as readily as the subject of Figure 3-2, with the same alacrity, in fact, as that with which most of our obese patients return to their usual and customary weight after weight loss.

This suggests that the heritable derangement of obesity may be an overriding disturbance at the level at which the central nervous system is set. This could be an exaggeration of those mechanisms to promote storage of energy which had survival value for our remote ancestors, but which in exaggerated form became a liability to us in our affluent society. If the fault truly lies with a derangement of central nervous system control, then the endocrine and other metabolic changes which we now associate with spontaneous obesity can develop secondary to the hyperphagia, and some of these in turn can contribute to perpetuating the obesity.

REFERENCES

1. Apfelbaum M, Bostsarron J, Lacatis D: Effect of caloric restriction and excessive caloric intake on energy expenditure. Am J Clin Nutr 24:1405-1409, 1971

2. Bray GA, Whipp BJ, Koyal S: Weight gain and work efficiency in normal volunteers (abstr). J Clin Invest 51:14a, 1972

3. Felig P, Horton ES, Runge CF, Sims EAH: Experimental obesity in man: Hyperaminoacidemia and diminished effectiveness of insulin in regulating peripheral amino acid release (abstr). Program of the 53rd Meeting, Endocrine Society, June 1971

4. Goldman, RF, Haisman, MF, Bynum G, Horton ES, Sims, EAH. Experimental Obesity in man VI. Metabolic Rate in relation to Dietary Intake. Proceedings of the Fogarty International Center Conference on obesity. 1973. In press.

5. Grey N, Kipnis DM: Effect of diet composition on the hyper-insulinemia of obesity. N Engl J Med 285:827-831, 1971

6. Hill FW: Nutrition Society Symposium. Energy costs of intermediate metabolism in intact animal. Fed Proc 30:1434-1473, 1971

7. Katch F, Michael ED, Horvath SM: Estimation of body volume by underwater weighing. Description of a simple method. J Appl Physiol 23:811, 1967

8. Miller DS, Mumford P, Stock MJ: Gluttony. II. Thermogenesis in overeating man. Am J Clin Nutr 20:1223-1229, 1967

9. Naeye RL, Roode P: The sizes and numbers of cells in visceral organs in human obesity. Am J Clin Path 54:251-253, 1970

10. Neumann RO: Experimentelle Beigräge zur Lehre von dem täglichen Nahrungsbedarf des Menschen unter besonderer Berücksichtigung der notwendigen Eiweifsmenge. Arch Hyg Bakteriol 45:1-87, 1902

11. O'Connell M, Danforth E Jr, Horton ES, Salans L, Sims EAH: Experimental obesity in man: III. Adrenocortical function. J Clin Endocrinol Metab. 36:323-329, 1973

12. Rabinowitz D, Zierler KL: Forearm metabolism in obesity and its response to intra-arterial insulin. Characterization of insulin resistance and evidence for adaptive hyperinsulinism. J Clin Invest 41:2173-2181, 1962

13. Salans, LB, Horton ES, Sims EAH: Experimental Obesity in man: Cellular Character of the adipose tissue. J Clin Invest 50:1005-1011, 1971

14. Sims EAH, Danforth E Jr, Horton ES, Bray GA, Glennon JA, Salans LB: Endocrine and metabolic effects of experimental obesity in man. Recent Progr Horm Res. In press

15. Sims EAH, Goldman RF, Gluck CM, Horton ES, Kelleher PC, Rowe DW: Experimental obesity in man. Trans Assoc Am Physicians 81:153-170, 1968

16. Sims EAH, Horton ES, Salans LB: Inducible metabolic abnormalities during development of obesity. Ann Rev Med 22:235-250, 1971

Starvation and the Behavior of the Obese

4

RICHARD E. NISBETT

Until quite recently, medical opinion on obesity could have been described approximately as follows: With a few exceptions due to obvious glandular or hormonal causes, obesity—that is, "simple" obesity—occurs without any apparent biologic cause other than caloric intake in excess of energy requirements. The strong implication of this view was that obesity represented an impairment of psychologic, if not, indeed, moral processes.

In contrast, the current mood is that the role played by biologic factors in "simple" obesity is very large, perhaps even fully determinative in the majority of instances. Although my own research began with a psychologic focus on the behavior of the obese, and although research has turned up a great many striking differences in the behavior of obese and normal-weight individuals, I have come increasingly to share the view that obesity is largely of biological origin. The behavioral differences between obese and

Much of the research reported here was supported by NSF Grant GB33918. An earlier version of this paper appeared in *Obesity and Bariatric Medicine,* 1:28-32, 1972.

normal individuals now seem to me to be secondary and, despite their potential medical importance, to lack any etiologic significance.

BIOLOGIC BASIS OF OBESITY

Obesity itself is in most cases largely the result of a "bad genetic draw." This conclusion stems in part from work by Hirsch and Knittle (12) and others (16) at Rockefeller University and by the Swedish physiologist Per Björntorp (2). Their work indicates that juvenile-onset obesity is the result of an elevated number and size of fat cells. Subjects with juvenile-onset obesity have been found to have as many as three times the number of fat cells as normal-weight individuals. In contrast, adult-onset obesity is associated with an increase in the size of fat cells but no increase in total number.

The importance of this work in understanding obesity becomes clear when it is realized that the number of fat cells in the adult is basically immutable. Dieting in adult humans can decrease the size of fat cells but has virtually no effect on the number of fat cells. After he loses weight, the formerly obese person is left with the same high number of fat cells to be refilled the moment will power fades. Conversely, overeating in the adult does not stimulate the growth of more fat cells. Prison volunteers paid by Dr. Sims to put on excess weight increased the size but not the number of their fat cells. This would seem to mean that persons who happen to have a large number of fat cells will in effect have a higher baseline of body fat. That is, constitutionally they are "programmed" to be fat.

The two factors that seem to influence the "fat baseline" are the individual's genetic make-up, and, perhaps also, his early nutritional experience. Strains of rats differ greatly in the percent of fat in their bodies and in their ability to gain weight on rich diets. (29) It seems likely that humans would show something approximating the genetic range that rats do. The actual data on parent-child similarity for obesity, though subject to interpretation on environmental grounds, show such a powerful relationship that it seems highly likely that heredity does play a role in human obesity. For example, one investigator (6) found that the slender parents in his sample *never* produced a fat child, while the very obese parents *never* produced a slender one.

The second factor that plays a likely role is early childhood nutrition. It is possible to affect the number of fat cells a rat will have as an adult during the first few weeks of life (16). It seems probable, although it has not yet been clearly demonstrated, that the fat baseline for humans could similarly be affected by overnutrition through the first few years of life.

The possibility of different genetic baselines for fat storage becomes important in view of the recent evidence suggesting that the body defends the adipose tissue mass. This appears to be done by hypothalamic feeding centers which adjust food intake to maintain fat stores at the baseline or "set point" level (25). If it is true that the hypothalamus defends the adipose tissue set point, then there seems to be no reason to assume that it defends the same set point in all individuals of the same height and bone structure. Instead, it is possible that the hypothalamus defends different baselines in different individuals, maintaining whatever set point the individual is favored with—or saddled with. This proposition suggests a new way of thinking about obesity. It would suggest that obesity, for some, is a "normal" or "ideal" body composition. Moreover, it would then follow that many individuals in the "overweight" population are actually "underweight." The person with a high set point for fat tissue will be under considerable social (and often medical) pressure to lose weight. If he does lose weight, his hypothalamus might be expected to respond to weight reduction in approximately the same way as the central nervous system of a leaner individual—with hunger. Such a person would, in effect, be starving all the time.

There are, in fact, many parallels between the behavior of obese humans and that of hungry humans and animals. Before describing the behavior of the obese, it will be helpful to describe in some detail the behavior changes that are induced by hunger. Some of these changes are familiar, but many of them are not widely known.

Behavior in Starvation

The food-deprived organism eats more when given the opportunity and eats more rapidly than the less deprived organism. The food-deprived organism is also more likely to eat in a new or strange setting, and so on. Less obvious are the effects of hunger on the response to the taste of food, which, until recently, had not been examined closely. Most researchers have simply assumed that the hungry organism is undiscriminating, eating large quantities of any available food without regard to its taste. This assumption now seems to be mistaken. The evidence, coming mostly from work by Jacobs and Sharma (14), suggests that the organism deprived of food consumes proportionally more good-tasting food and proportionally less bad-tasting food than does the less deprived one.

Jacobs and Sharma (14) offered dogs and rats either standard laboratory chow, chow with improved flavor due to the addition of fats or saccharin, or chow which had been made to taste bad through addition of quinine or cellulose. Animals were either allowed to eat whenever they wanted or were given only one brief meal in every 24 hours. *Ad lib* and deprived animals consumed equivalent amounts of standard chow, but deprived animals consumed much more good-tasting chow than *ad lib* animals and consumed much less bad-tasting chow. The evidence thus suggests that the deprived animal becomes increasingly more responsive to taste, consuming proportionally more good-tasting food and less bad-tasting food. Additional supportive work has been done by Gross (11), who subjected young rats, for a period of weeks, to deprivation schedules that were so severe they could not maintain normal weight. When returned to *ad lib* conditions, these animals rejected cellulose-diluted chow relatively more than did animals always maintained on *ad lib* schedules, and consumed relatively more chow to which fats had been added than did the always-*ad lib* animals.

Hunger also has powerful effects on other kinds of behavior. Most of what we know about the effects of extreme hunger on general behavior comes from the classic World War II work of Keys, *et al.* (15). Their subjects were conscientious objectors who volunteered to lose 24% of their body weight over a 24-week period. This was done by restricting the mens' daily caloric intake to approximately 1600 Cal while requiring them to continue normal work routines. During the course of this regimen, the subjects showed three chief symptoms: They became progressively more prone to emotional upset, more apathetic and inactive, and less interested in sex.

Irritability was quite marked throughout semistarvation and outbursts of temper were so frequent that the group meetings held during the control period had to be stopped. Periods of elation also occurred, which were inevitably followed by periods of depression. Psychological tests revealed progressively more emotional upset and pathology as semi-starvation proceeded.

Activity of any kind was aversive to the men. They preferred to sit and do nothing than to perform any kind of formerly pleasurable work or play. This lack of *joie de vivre* extended to sex. Many engagements were broken, few of the men continued to date, and masturbation and nocturnal emission virtually ceased.

The Behavior of Obese Humans

Although almost none of the research on obese humans seems to have been guided by the hypothesis that the obese are hungry, it is fair to say that the major areas in which obese humans have been shown to differ behaviorally from normal-weight humans parallel almost exactly the areas affected by hunger. Most of the data we have on the behavior of obese humans comes from a program initiated in 1965 by Stanley Schachter and his colleagues (27, 28), at Columbia University. In this research program, the "obese" subjects were usually college students whose weight was 15% or more over the average for their height. The average obese subject in the series was about 30% overweight. Extensive reviews of this research have been published (20, 21, 27), and will be described here only briefly.

Like the hungry organism, the obese human eats more at a given sitting and eats more rapidly (27). The obese person also has a greater readiness to eat, as indicated by the fact that in a novel environment containing food, he is more likely to eat than is the normal individual (26). And like the hungry organism, the obese individual is highly taste responsive, eating extra-large portions of good food and unusually small portions of bad food (19, 20).

The eating behavior of the obese seems to reflect a constant, moderately strong degree of hunger, and is affected remarkably little by the physiologic cues that increase or reduce the normal individual's interest in food. In one experiment, Schachter *et al.* (28) asked obese and normal subjects to "taste" a variety of crackers. Some of their subjects had just eaten two roast beef sandwiches and some had eaten nothing for several hours. Normal subjects, to no one's surprise, ate fewer crackers in the tasting session if they had just eaten two sandwiches than they did if food-deprived. Overweight subjects, however, ate just as many crackers if they had eaten the sandwiches as they did if deprived. Similarly, I have found that self-report of hunger varies with the deprivation state for normal subjects but does not vary for obese subjects (Fig. 4-1) (19). In

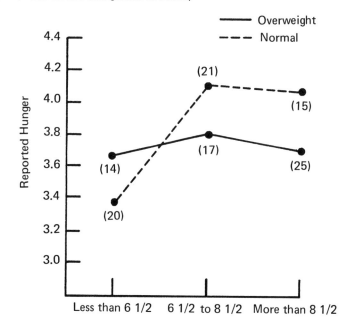

Hours of Deprivation

Fig. 4-1. Hunger reports of obese and normal subjects as a function of number of hours of food deprivation. (Nisbett RE: Taste, deprivation and weight determinants of eating behavior. J Pers Soc Psychol 10:107-116, 1968)

another study (22) in a supermarket, normal-weight individuals did more and more impulse buying as their state of food deprivation increased, whereas overweight shoppers did a moderate amount of impulse buying regardless of their state of deprivation. It is as if the long-term hunger of the obese completely overrides the physiologic cues associated with short-term changes in nutritional state.

The obese seem markedly similar to the starving subjects of Keys et al. (15) in a variety of other behavioral areas. Overweight humans appear to be more prone to emotional upset than normal-weight individuals. Schachter et al. (28) found that overweight subjects are more frightened by the prospect of receiving electric shocks than are normal subjects. Schachter (27) reports that Rodin found the proof-reading and monitoring performance of obese subjects deteriorated when they listened to emotionally charged tapes, while the performance of normal subjects did not suffer. The greater emotionality of the obese is reflected in the scores they receive on psychological adjustment batteries. Moore *et al.* (18) reanalyzed the data collected in a mental health survey of a random sample of midtown Manhattan residents. The obese individuals in that sample were found to be more emotionally disturbed by a variety of indicators. Interestingly, respondents from lower socioeconomic groups were more obese than the respondents from higher status. Perhaps people of lower socioeconomic status are subjected to less social and/or medical pressure to lose weight. If so, it might be that more of them are at their baseline for body weight and that the overweight persons of the middle and upper class are primarily the ones who are struggling to keep their weight down and hence are suffering the consequent emotional disorders. To test this hypothesis, I have reexamined the data from the Midtown survey and found that, almost exclusively, the overweight members of the middle and upper socioeconomic group are the ones who show excessive symptoms of emotional distress.

If it is correct that the emotional distress of many overweight people is due to the fact that they are actually "underweight," then any systematic attempts at weight loss ought to result in further deterioration. This is a terribly important point, yet the data on this issue are contradictory and incomplete. Some investigators (3, 8, 9, 31) do report deterioration, often severe, including depression, irritability and even psychosis and attempted suicide. Other investigators, however, report no untoward effects. It is possible, of course, that the different results reflect the use of different patient populations. The untoward effects may have been obtained from patients already below their baselines, and the less deleterious results may have been obtained with patients at, or even perhaps above, their baselines at the start of treatment. Further systematic research on this point, with a view toward the discovery of good predictor variables, is badly needed.

The other symptoms of hunger reported by Keys *et al.* (15) also seem to be present in the obese. Mayer and his colleagues find the obese to be highly inactive, even remaining relatively immobile when engaging in "active" sports. Chirico and Stunkard (5) find that, within given occupational roles, the obese individual manages to walk much less during the course of his day than the normal individual. Many investigations have found that the obese report that they spend unusually large amounts of time in the most highly sedentary of pursuits—e.g., listening to the radio or watching television.

Sexual interest has not been well studied to date, but the psychoanalyst Hilde Bruch (3) reports that her obese patients as a group have remarkably little sexual interest. In a preliminary unpublished investigation, I have found that obese male college students have fewer orgasms than normal students. This finding also obtains for the number of nocturnal orgasms, which of course would be little influenced by social considerations.

FREE FATTY ACIDS AND OBESITY

It is clear, then, that the obese person and the hungry individual have much in common. These similarities raise the question of whether there are also physiological indications that the obese are hungry. The answer appears to be yes. The most generally agreed upon physiological index of hunger is the level of free fatty acids (FFA) in the blood. When the organism is food-deprived (or is cold or exercises), FFA are mobilized from adipose tissue to meet energy requirements. When something is eaten, FFA levels fall rapidly.

Many studies show that the FFA level is higher in obese persons than in normal people (10). It has usually been presumed that this elevation of FFA in the blood of the obese was simply due to the elevation of fat stores which essentially "spill over" into the bloodstream. It does not seem likely, however, that high levels of FFA are simply an artifact of large fat deposits. On occasion, investigators have found no elevation of FFA levels in their obese patients. In these instances, the investigators were working with obese patients who had been overeating and gaining weight during the period immediately preceding the tests. More importantly, when the obese person loses weight, FFA's increase still further (7, 13, 17).*

An extremely important fact about FFA level for present concerns is that, in the obese, it is relatively inflexible, showing little variation in response to short-term nutritional changes (10). During a day's fast, FFA

*Dr. Sims' important work on experimentally induced obesity is obviously quite pertinent here. Unfortunately, the results for FFA are not consistent. In an earlier sample Sims *et al.* (30) found no elevation of FFA in fattened prisoners. In a second sample, of subjects in whom dietary intake was controlled, there does appear to be an elevation.

levels of the obese increase only slightly or not at all. Normal subjects, in contrast, start with low levels, and in approximately 20-24 hours' deprivation their levels of FFA equal those found in the obese. The FFA response of the obese to ingestion of food is also sluggish. During a fast, the levels of FFA in normal subjects drop quickly to nonfasting levels when they drink 50-100 g glucose. The FFA response of obese subjects is both slower and less complete than that of normals (10).

The physiological data are in agreement, then, with the behavioral data. Overweight individuals behave as if their hunger switch were stuck in the "on" position. They eat more at a given sitting, they eat more rapidly, they are more responsive to taste, and neither their eating behavior, their self-report of hunger, nor even the attractiveness of supermarket food is much affected by short-term changes in the state of deprivation. The physiological evidence justifies this inflexibly hungry pattern: FFA level is inflexibly high.

HUNGER, OBESITY, AND THE VENTROMEDIAL HYPOTHALAMUS

There are good reasons to believe that the behavioral effects of hunger are mediated at least in part by the ventromedial hypothalamus (VMH). Electrophysiological evidence indicates that the VMH is quite well attuned to the nutritional state of the animal, showing activity when the animal is well fed and showing inactivity when the animal is not well fed (1, 23). Secondly, Pfaff (24) has shown that if you compare a well-fed animal with an animal which has been held to a very restricted diet for 7 days or so, you find shrinking of the nucleoli of the cells in the VMH of the deprived animal. This indicates that a kind of functional lesion of the VMH occurs with food deprivation. Thirdly, there is the large body of literature describing the effects of electrolytic lesion of the VMH. The behavioral syndrome is a familiar one: An animal with a VMH lesion eats more per meal, eats more rapidly, is more likely to eat in strange surroundings, and is hyperresponsive to the taste of its food (27).

The effects of the VMH lesion are not restricted to eating behavior. The animal is quite emotional by all existing indicators of that sort of thing in a rat. It has long been known to be extremely irritable and will fly into a rage in response to the normal routine of handling in the laboratory.

Recently, it has been shown that the animal with a VMH lesion is also quite fearful. It has a lower threshold for flinching and jumping in response to electric shock, and it learns more quickly to avoid electric shock than the normal animal. Finally, it is very inactive both in its home cage and in an activity wheel, and it is also hyposexual. The parallels to hunger and to the behavior of the obese human seem too marked to be coincidental. It seems quite likely that the VMH is deeply involved in the phenomena seen in starvation and obesity.

CLINICAL IMPLICATIONS

Mechanisms aside, what are the implications for practitioners in the field of obesity? There is a very real possibility that some people are overweight because they have eaten themselves above their set points. There can be no very great direct utility of the present facts for individual practice until much more is known on that subject than at present. It seems clear that there are some very direct implications for clinical research. Some way of diagnosing the "baseline" or ideal weight for each individual is needed. Some clues as to how this diagnosis might be achieved are already available in the research to date. Particularly promising is the prospect of using the size and number of fat cells. Ultimately, it may be possible to predict the chances of success in dieting and to estimate the likelihood that the patient will suffer loss of emotional stability, activity drive, and sexual interest.

Unfortunately we do not now have good predictive tools, and there is at present no way to diagnose the "set point" of a particular patient. Perhaps, however, it is desirable for the practitioner to reflect available knowledge to his patients in the form of a cautionary statement. One physician, who is familiar with the evidence I have described, has written the following note to me:

> I have for years tried to get the point across to my patients before they start to lose weight that they need to make an intelligent decision. For some it may be better to accept the social and health risks of obesity, whatever they are, and go ahead and enjoy the pleasures of eating. I point out to them that if they undertake to lose weight and maintain a normal weight, they will never again be able to eat as they have been eating at their obese weight. They must

be made to realize that they will be in a sense dietary cripples. They will never be able to eat freely of their foods as their normal-weight counterparts do and maintain their new normal weight. I also point out this is not fair, but neither is it fair to be born blind or with other physical abnormalities. For some time, the pain of maintaining a normal weight is not counterbalanced by the benefits of being at a "normal" weight. I see little reason to attempt to coerce these people into doing so.

REFERENCES

1. Anand GK, Chhina GS, and Singh B: Effect of glucose on the activity of hypothalamic "feeding centers." Science 138:597-598, 1962

2. Björntrop P: Disturbances in the regulation of food intake. Adv Psychosom Med 1972.

3. Bruch H: The Importance of Overweight. New York, W. W. Norton, 1957

4. Bullen BA, Reed RB, Mayer J: Physical activity of obese and nonobese adolescent girls appraised by motion picture sampling. Am J Clin Nutr 14:211-223, 1964

5. Chirico A, Stunkard AJ: Physical activity and human obesity. N Engl J Med 263:935-940, 1960

6. Davenport CB: Body-build and its inheritance. Carnegie Institute of Washington, Pub. 329, 1923

7. Genuth SM: Effects of prolonged fasting on insulin secretions. Diabetes 15:798-806, 1966

8. Gluckman ML, Hirsch J: The response of obese patients to weight reduction. Psychosom Med 30:1-11, 1968

9. Gluckman ML, Hirsch J, McGully RS, Barron BA, Knittle JL: The response of obese patients to weight reduction. Psychosom Med 30:359-373, 1968

10. Gordon ES: Metabolic aspects of obesity, Advances in Metabolic Disorders, Edited by R Levine and R Left. New York, Academic Press, 1970

11. Gross LP: Scarcity, unpredictability and eating behavior in rats. Unpublished PhD dissertation, Columbia University, 1968

12. Hirsch J, Knittle JL: Cellularity of obese and nonobese human adipose tissue. Fed Proc 29:1516-1521, 1970

13. Issekutz B, Bortz WM, Miller HI, Wroldsen A: Plasma free fatty acid response to exercise in obese humans. Metabolism 16:492-502, 1967

14. Jacobs HL, Sharma KN: Taste versus calories: sensory and metabolic signals in the control of food intake. Ann NY Acad Sci 157:1084-1125, 1969

15. Keys A, Brôzek J, Henschel A, Mickelsen O, Taylor HL: The Biology of Human Starvation. Minneapolis, Univ Minnesota Press, 1950

16. Knittle JL, Hirsch J: Effect of early nutrition on the development of rat epididymal fat pads: Cellularity and metabolism. J Clin Invest 47:2091, 1968

17. Liebermeister H, Daweke H, Gries FA, Schilling WH, Grüneklee D, Probst G, Jahnke K: Einflüss der Gewichtsreduktion auf Metabolite des Kohlenhydrat-und Fettstoffwechsels und auf das Verhalten des Seruminsulins bei Adopösitas. Diabetologia 4:123-132, 1968

18. Moore ME, Stunkard A, Srole L: Obesity, social class, and mental illness. JAMA 000:138-142, 1962

19. Nisbett RE: Taste, deprivation and weight determinants of eating behavior. J Pers Soc Psychol 10:107-116, 1968

20. Nisbett RE: Eating behavior and obesity in men and animals. Adv Psychosom Med 7:173-193, 1972

21. Nisbett RE: Hunger, obesity and the ventromedial hypothalamus. Psych Rev 79:433-453, 1972

22. Nisbett RE, Kanouse DE: Obesity, food deprivation, and supermarket shopping behavior. J Pers Soc Psychol 12:289-294, 1969

23. Oomura Y, Ooyama H, Naka F, Yamamoto T, Ono T, Kobayashi N: Some stochastical patterns of single unit discharges in the cat hypothalamus under chronic conditions. Ann NY Acad Sci 157:666-689, 1969

24. Pfaff DW: Histological differences between ventromedial hypothalamic neurones of well fed and underfed rats. Nature (Lond) 223:77-78, 1969

25. Powley TL, Keesey R: Relationships of body weight to the lateral hypothalamic feeding syndrome. J Comp Physiol Psychol 70:25-36, 1970

26. Ross L: Cue- and cognition-controlled eating among obese and normal subjects. Unpublished PhD Dissertation, Columbia University, New York, 1969

27. Schachter S: Some extraordinary facts about obese humans and rats. Am Psychol 26:129-144, 1971

28. Schachter S, Goldman R, Gordon A: Effects of fear, food deprivation and obesity on eating. J Pers Soc Psychol 10:107-116, 1968

29. Schemmel R, Mickelsen O, Gill JL: Dietary obesity in rats: body weight and body fat accretion in seven strains of rats. J Nutr 100:1041-1048, 1970

30. Sims EA, Kelleher PE, Horton ES, Gluck CM, Goodman RF, Rowe DA: Experimental obesity in man. Excerpta Med Monogr 1968

31. Stunkard AJ: The "dieting depression." Am J Med 000:77-86, 1957

SOME CLINICAL ASPECTS OF OBESITY

II

The Varieties of Obesity

5

GEORGE A. BRAY

Obesity, like high blood pressure, is not a disease; it is a symptom. It represents one visible consequence of ingesting more calories than are being utilized. A number of attempts have been made to classify obesities. One of the most widely used classifications is that of von Noorden who popularized "exogenous" and "endogenous" obesity (45). The former group is composed of patients whose obesity appears to result directly from the ingestion of excess food. Endogenous obesity, on the other hand, includes the various endocrinopathies associated with corpulence. With advancing knowledge about the mechanisms controlling food intake, newer approaches to the classification of obesity have become possible (6, 33, 43). We will discuss two of these: (1) an anatomic classification based on the number of adipocytes and (2) an etiologic classification.

ANATOMIC CLASSIFICATION–HYPERTROPHIC VS. HYPERPLASTIC OBESITY

The accumulation of body fat can occur in one of two ways: by storing excess triglyceride in adipocytes which already exist (hypertrophy) or by increasing the number of adipocytes (hyperplasia). It is conceivable that the stimulus of increased caloric intake could evoke production of new fat cells with an augmentation in their total number (40) (Table 5-1). In one study, Bjurlf (5) examined this question by measuring the size, thickness, and number of fat cells in adipose tissue of 60 males at autopsy. The size of the fat cells was correlated with body weight, reflecting differences in nutrition. The number of fat cells, on the other hand, was related to the thickness of the subcutaneous fat. He concluded that the genetic factors in obesity were reflected mainly in the number of adipocytes.

This basic concept of hypertrophic and hyperplastic obesity has been confirmed and amplified by the use of more elegant techniques developed by Hirsch and Gallian (26) and by Sjostrom *et al.* (50) and is reviewed in chapter 2 of this volume. These investigators have clearly shown that all fat people have enlarged adipocytes (4, 8, 28, 48) and thus all obesity is "hypertrophic" from the anatomic viewpoint. Most patients with juvenile-onset obesity have, in addition, an increased number of fat cells (4, 8, 28, 48). Thus two groups are defined; those with a normal total number of fat cells and a second group with an increased total number of fat cells (Table 5-1).

ETIOLOGIC CLASSIFICATION OF OBESITY

An etiologic classification can be developed from studies of experimental animals. In the experimental animal, obesity can be produced in at least five different ways (Table 5-1) (9): (1) hypothalamic injury, (2) endocrine manipulation, (3) dietary manipulation, (4) restriction of physical activity, and (5) genetic transmission.

Hypothalamic Obesity

Hypothalamic injuries that induce obesity can be produced with at least three different approaches. The most widely used experimental technique is the introduction of bilateral electrolytic injury in the ventromedial region of the hypothalamus. Careful mapping of this area has indicated that the most effective lesions are those in the lower anterior portion of the ventromedial nucleus (52). In addition, hypothalamic insult by microsurgical cuts in the fiber tracts leading from this ventromedial

Table 5-1. Classification of Obesity in Experimental Animals

Etiologic	Anatomic
Hypothalamic injury	Hypertrophic
Electrolytic	
Microsurgical	
Chemical	
Endocrine	Hypertrophic
Excess corticosteroids	
Hyperinsulinism	
Castration	
Dietary	Hypertrophic
Gorging	↓
High-fat diet	? Hyperplastic
Inactivity	Hypertrophic
Genetic transmission	
Dominant inheritance (A^{iy}, A^{vy}, A^{y})	Hypertrophic
Recessive inheritance (ob, db, db/ad, fa)	Hyperplastic
Polygenic	?

nucleus (32) or chemical injury with gold thioglucose (10), piperidyl mustard (47), monosodium glutamate (46), or nitro-quinoline-1-oxide (56), all induce obesity. The experimental picture produced in animals with these lesions depends upon the extent and location of the injury (52).

Prior to the lesion, the activity pattern and estrus cycles are regular (11). Food intake and body weight are constant. Following an electrolytic injury to the ventromedial nucleus, the estrous cycles become irregular and unpredictable. Food intake increases sharply and may rise twofold. The increased food intake and decreased physical activity lead to a "dynamic phase" with progressive weight gain. Metabolic rate is normal or slightly diminished. After a period of continually increased food intake, body weight reaches a new plateau, with a "static phase" of obesity and a fall in food intake. If the obese rat with a hypothalamic lesion is fasted, it loses weight; as soon as it has access to food, however, the animal regains weight to the same or a slightly higher level than the one at which fasting began (37). Thus, the introduction of a hypothalamic lesion has altered the set point at which body weight can be regulated. Weight gain after hypothalamic injury is an example of hypertrophic obesity; that is, in these animals there is an enlargement of individual adipocytes with no increase in the total number of fat cells (27).

Studies of the endocrine and metabolic alterations in these animals with injuries of the hypothalamus have revealed several interesting facts. First, the glucose concentration in plasma is unaltered in the obese animal (18). Second, the pattern of individual fatty acid stored in fat changes with an increase in the quantity of unsaturated acids (palmitic) and a decrease in the unsaturated fatty acids (22). Third, the obese animals are hyperinsulinemic (18). This was suggested by finding hypertrophy of the beta cells in the islets of Langerhans (38) and has been confirmed by direct measurements of plasma insulin (18, 23). The hyperinsulinemia occurs promptly after injury to the hypothalamus if food intake is allowed but does not occur if all food is removed (19). Thus, the stimulus of food intake leads to an exaggerated output of insulin from the pancreatic beta cells of rats with hypothalamic injury. In spite of hyperinsulinemia, the rat with hypothalamic obesity does not become hypoglycemic but, rather, maintains normal blood sugar. This could occur either because peripheral clearance of glucose was reduced or because glucose production was increased. The removal of glucose has been measured and is normal or increased (20). Moreover, the muscle and adipose tissues of rats with hypothalamic obesity are normally sensitive to insulin. It thus appears that in hypothalamic obesity, glucose production must be enhanced, but the mechanism for this is unclear.

Endocrine Abnormalities and Obesity

Three different endocrine manipulations can produce obesity: (1) administration of insulin (29), (2) administration of glucocorticoids (30), and (3) castration (55). Animals which become obese if insulin is injected daily will return to normal weight if the injections of insulin are stopped. Although insulin-treated rats are hyperphagic, the mechanisms are unclear. Two possibilities need to be considered. The first is that insulin acts to produce hyperphagia indirectly by lowering blood sugar. The second possibility is that it acts directly on the brain to increase or modulate feeding activity. At present the evidence showing that insulin has a direct effect on the brain is limited. However, insulin does influence the feeding center indirectly. The lateral hypothalamus is the area involved in the control of food-seeking behavior, and injury to this area produces a phagia. If such animals are carefully nursed so that they do not die, food-seeking behavior will return in a modified form (54). Increased food intake in rats that have recovered from lateral hypothalamic lesions will occur in response to cold but not in response to hypoglycemia. One might thus suspect that hypoglycemia was the major mechanism by which insulin stimulates food intake (15).

Administration of glucocorticoids will also increase the quantity of body fat. In many experiments, total body weight does not increase even though steroid administration modifies the metabolism of adipose tissue toward increased fat storage (30).

Castration is a third endocrine manipulation which will lead to substantial redistribution of body fat (55). This is understandable in view of the effects of reproductive hormones, particularly estrogens, on the distribution of body fat. However, neither corticosteroids nor estrogens will cause the degree of obesity that can be produced by hypothalamic injury or by the injection of insulin.

Dietary Manipulation

Manipulation of the diet can produce obesity in one of two ways. The first is to convert animals which normally eat frequent meals into animals which eat meals only one or two times a day (16). If rats in one group are allowed to eat *ad libitum* and rats in the second group are fed an identical quantity of food by stomach tube twice a day, the content of body fat in the tube-fed rats will be significanlty greater than in the animals fed *ad libitum* (14). Present evidence indicates that animals which eat food rapidly and, therefore, have few meals tend to convert a larger fraction of the calories to fat with increased nitrogen excretion. The rapid ingestion of calories enhances the output of insulin, which is in turn lipogeneic. In animals that eat many small meals, the quantity of calories stored as fat is reduced.

An increase in the quantity of fat in the diet is a second mechanism that produces obesity in certain strains of rats (49). When dietary fat is increased, rats are unable to reduce their total food intake to compensate for the increased caloric density. Increased fat accumulates by enlargement of adipocytes and the animals become grossly obese. The reason for the failure to compensate for increased caloric density is unclear. Fat-induced obesity, like hypothalamic injury and endocrine manipulation, is a hypertrophic form of obesity with little or no hyperplasia of fat depots (Table 5-1).

Restricted Activity

The fourth method for producing experimental obesity is by restriction of physical activity (31). Mayer *et al.* (44) have graphically demonstrated this phenomenon (Fig. 5-1). In their study, rats were exercised up to 8 hours per day. Food intake was proportional to energy expenditure when activity ranged between 1 and 5.5 hours per day. When forced activity was longer than this or less than 1 hour, however, food intake compensated inappropriately. At the higher levels of work output, food intake could not match energy needs and the animals lost weight. At very low levels of energy output, however, both food intake and body weight increased. This is a fascinating observation that requires additional experimental study. It suggests that at low levels of physical activity food intake may paradoxically increase.

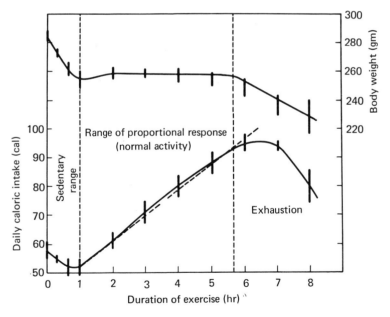

Fig. 5-1. Effect of activity on food intake. Food intake and body weight were measured during intervals of activity from less than to more than 8 hours per day. (Mayer J, Marshall NB, Vitale JJ, Christensen JH, Moshagekhi MB, Stare FJ: Exercise, food intake and body weight in normal rats and genetically obese adult mice. Am J Physiol 177:544-548, 1954)

Genetic Obesity

The final variety of experimental obesity is that transmitted genetically (9). Among experimental animals, a number of forms of obesity are transmitted in this way. They include obesity in the yellow mouse, which is transmitted by an autosomal dominant, and obesity in three strains of mice (obese, adipose, and diabetes), transmitted as an autosomal mendelian recessive. Obesity is also observed in inbred strains such as the New Zealand obese mouse (NZO) or the Japanese KK mouse and in certain varieties of desert rodents that become obese when their diet is changed from vegetables and green leafy plants to laboratory chow.

Several of the genetically transmitted forms of obesity have hyperplasia of their fat depots (35). Johnson *et al.* (35) have shown that the "obese" mouse (ob/ob) and the fatty rat (fa/fa) (34) both have increased total numbers of adipocytes. These two models thus reflect genetically transmitted defects manifested by increased numbers of adipose cells.

The genetically transmitted forms of obesity have a number of characteristics in common (9). All animals are hyperphagic—that is, they all eat more food than lean controls. Food intake may be only slightly elevated, but in some instances it may increase more than twofold. The fat animal is usually inactive compared to his lean litter mate. Hyperglycemia of varying degrees is present in most of the mice but is not present routinely in the fatty rat. All animals, however, are hyperinsulinemic, with values in some animals reaching very high levels indeed. Insulin resistance (*i.e.,* a diminished response to the administration of exogenous insulin) is present in many of these forms of obesity but can be overcome by two mechanisms: (1) decreasing body weight (3) and (2) damaging the pancreatic islets with alloxan or streptozotocin (42). At present there is no clear biochemical basis for explaining the obesity in any of these animals. The hypothalamus, the adipose tissue, and the pancreas with abnormal insulin production or secretion have been the principal sights toward which scientific activity has been focused (9).

THE VARIETIES OF HUMAN OBESITY

By analogy with the forms of experimental obesity, etiologic mechanisms for human obesity can be divided into several categories: (1)

hypothalamic obesity, (2) endocrine obesity, (3) physical inactivity, (4) dietary obesity, (5) genetic obesity, and (6) drug-induced obesity (28) (Table 5-2).

There is clear evidence dating from the work of Babinski (2) and Fröhlich (17) at the turn of the century that injury to the hypothalamus can produce obesity. Over the ensuing years, a hundred or more such cases have been described (7). We have had the chance to study 6 such patients in whom obesity was clearly associated with an anatomically defined lesion in the hypothalamus. The diagnosis was different in each of our patients.

One developed her obesity at a young age, in association with a dermoid cyst of the third ventricle. When brought to our hospital at 6 months of age, she was already obese. Her weight rose sharply after the initial operation and remained consistently above the 97th percentile. Her

Table 5-2.   Classification of Obesity in Man

Etiologic	Anatomic
Hypothalamic	Hypertrophic
Tumors	
Solid (Fröhlich-Babinski syndrome)	
Leukemia	
Inflammatory	
Traumatic	
Increased intracranial pressure (empty sella, pseudotumor cerebri)	
Endocrine	Hypertrophic
Cushing's disease	
Insulinoma	
Castration	
Stein-Levinthal syndrome	
Pregnancy	
Inactivity	Hypertrophic
Genetic	
Juvenile onset	Hyperplastic
Laurence-Moon-Biedl syndrome	?
Hyperostosis frontalis interna	
Alstrom's syndrome	
Prader-Willi syndrome	
Drugs	
Phenothiazines	Hypertrophic (?)
Estrogens	
Cyproheptadine	
Essential	

weight has continued to rise and at her last visit at age 14 she weighed in excess of 250 lb.

The second patient was found to have a chordoma at the base of the clivus. Chordomas are tumors arising from the embryologic notochord (41). In the adult the residum of this tissue is found in the nucleus pulposis of the intervertebral disc. Occasionally chordomas become malignant. Most such tumors are observed in the region of the coccyx, but about a third of them are intracranial. Their usual symptoms are those of intracranial tumor; our patient is the only reported case with obesity.

Our third patient had a lipoma of the interpeduncular fossa. The fourth had a craniopharyngioma (53). This tumor developing from the embryologic remnants along the stalk of the hypothseal duct is the commonest cause of hypothalamic obesity in man. In our series, however, there was only one patient with this problem.

The only man in our series had an aneurysm of the internal carotid artery, which had been clipped prior to our seeing him. Following the insertion of the clip, he gained 100 lb in a 6-month period. Prior to that time, his weight had been constant at less than 160 lb. Our final patient had a meningioma of the right optic nerve.

Patients with hypothalamic obesity are rare. In a review of the literature, we have found 68 cases in addition to ours, in whom enough data was reported for analysis of their weight gain. The weight distribution among the 68 patients is shown in Table 5-3. Most patients with hypothalamic obesity developed their problem before 40 years of age. Only 9 of the 68 were over 40 years old. The major source of pathology in these patients was a craniopharyngioma, with other lesions being much less common. In our patients, the evidence suggests that most of the obesity

Table 5-3. Age Distribution Among Cases with Hypothalamic Obesity

Age	No. of cases
0–10	6
11–20	14
21–30	20
31–40	16
41–50	7
51–60	4
61–70	1
	68

occurred by hypertrophy of the fat cells, although in one patient, it was possible that hyperplasia had developed, too. In addition to obesity, all patients had one or more additional symptoms (Table 5-4). Headache, visual impairment, and abnormalities of the reproductive system (amenorrhea in women, loss of libido in men, and failure of sexual development in children) were the most common associated symptoms. Polyuria, polydipsia, diabetes insipidus, somnolence, and behavior disorders were also reported but with considerably lower frequency. Thus, hypothalamic obesity in man, when it occurs, is invariably associated with other manifestations of intracranial disease.

The distribution of body weight among these patients shows the following pattern. There were no patients weighing over 300 lb in whom a hypothalamic lesion was clearly the cause of their obesity (Table 5-5). Indeed, there were only two weighing between 275 and 300 lb. It is thus clear that in patients weighing over 250 lb the obesity is rarely based on hypothalamic injury. Gross obesity of the hyperplastic kind, which develops in early life, is thus unlikely to be the result of a primary hypothalamic lesion. In addition to the relatively limited total body weight, none of the patients gained more than 125 lb. We can summarize by saying that hypothalamic obesity in man is a hypertrophic form of the disease associated with increased food intake and with weight gain.

A second form of obesity, the syndrome of polycystic ovaries described by Stein and Leventhal, is a combination of hypothalamic and endocrine obesity (21). This complex of hypo- or amenorrhea, of moderate hirsutism and weight gain usually develops in young women shortly after menarche. They are often infertile. Menstruation and fertility frequently can be restored by wedge resection of the ovary. These women show increased

Table 5-4.   Frequency of Symptoms in 68 Patients with Hypothalamic Obesity Due to Tumors

	No.	%
Headache	42	62
Visual impairment	49	72
Reproductive symptoms	44	65
Polyuria and/or polydipsia	23	34
Somnolence	31	46
Behavior disorders	8	12
Convulsions	3	4

Table 5-5. Distribution of Body Weight Among Patients with Hypothalamic
           Obesity

Maximal wt	No. of cases
100–125	4
126–150	13
151–175	9
176–200	10
201–225	9
226–250	1
251–275	1
Over 276	1

adrenal and ovarian function which, along with the hyperphagia and weight gain, suggests a hypothalamic variety of obesity. There is, however, little data to support this concept.

The second broad form of obesity, analogous to that seen in experimental animals, is that induced by endocrine abnormality. The most striking forms of endocrine obesity in human subjects are seen in patients with Cushing's syndrome (51). This illness can result from hyperplasia of the adrenal gland or from excess secretion of corticosteroids from an adrenal adenoma or an adrenal carcinoma. It is accompanied by a characteristic pattern of weight gain. Fat is usually accumulated in the trunk, in the supraclavicular fossa, and in the posterior cervical region. Arms and legs are generally spared. Hypertension, abnormalities in glucose tolerance, and abnormalities in adrenal function are characteristic of this syndrome. The basis for the accumulation of excess fat is unclear but may well reflect alterations in insulin secretion which occur in these people.

Hyperinsulinism is a second form of endocrine abnormality that can produce obesity in humans (36). In the adult-onset form of diabetes, weight gain frequently precedes or is associated with the onset of hyperinsulinism. If the excess weight is lost, the impairment in glucose tolerance and the hyperinsulinemia revert towards normal. It appears likely, however, that the increased weight is associated with the pathogenesis of adult-onset diabetes.

Insulinomas are a second mechanism for hyperinsulinism. In persons with tumors producing excess quantities of insulin, there is often an associated weight gain, though it is usually limited to less than 20 lb.

Inactivity is a major factor in human obesity (12, 13). There is clear evidence that physical activity is decreasing as our society becomes more mechanized. There is evidence also from epidemiologic studies to suggest that, as economic status improves, inactivity frequently increases and obesity results. Similarly, people who have been accustomed to high levels of activity, particularly athletes, frequently undergo substantial weight gain when their life pattern adjusts from the activity of an athletic career to the inactivity of most sedentary occupations.

The genetic forms of obesity in man are less clearly defined than in experimental animals. Present evidence suggests that the hyperplastic forms of obesity in man may well be genetic (5). In addition, three other varieties of human obesity may be genetically transmitted. The first of these is the Laurence-Moon-Bardet-Biedl (LMBB) (39) syndrome, a rare form of disease with retinal abnormalities, polydactilism, mental retardation, and obesity (Table 5-6). A syndrome described by Alstrom *et al.* (54) is similar in some respects to the LMBB syndrome, but differs in several important features (Table 5-6). The so-called Prader-Willi syndrome (24) characterized by hypotonia, mental deficiency, hypogonadism, and obesity may also be genetically transmitted. Hyperostosis frontalis interna (the Morgagni-Morel Syndrome) is also a genetic disease in which obesity is a significant feature (25), but the underlying mechanisms for this and the other diseases are poorly understood and await the results of future research.

Table 5-6. A Comparison of Some Features of Three Syndromes with Obesity

| Manifestation | Syndrome | | |
	Prader-Willi	LMBB[a]	Alstrom
Obesity	Gross	Yes	Yes
Mental Status	Retarded	Retarded	Normal
Vision	Normal	Retinitis pigmentosa	Atypical retinal degeneration
Gonads	Hypogenital	Hypogenital	Normal
Deafness	No	Rare	Yes
Diabetes mellitus	No	No	Yes
Muscles	Hypotonia	Normal	Normal
Hand	—	Polydactyly	—

[a] Laurence-Moon-Bardet-Biedl syndrome.

REFERENCES

1. Alstrom DH, Hallgreen B, Nilsson LB, Asander H: Retinal degeneration combined with obesity, diabetes mellitus and neurogenous deafness. Acta Psychiatr Scand 34:(Suppl 129)1-35, 1959

2. Babinski MJ: Tumeur du corps pituitaire sans acromegalie et avec le developpement des organes genitaux. Rev Neurol 8:531-533, 1900

3. Batt RAL, Miahle P: Insulin resistance of the inherently obese mouse—obob. Nature (Lond) 212:289-290, 1966

4. Bjorntorp P, Sjostrom L: Number and size of adipose tissue fat cells in relation to metabolism in human obesity. Metabolism 20:703-713, 1971

5. Bjurlf P: Atherosclerosis and body-build with special reference to size and number of subcutaneous fat cells. Acta Med Scand [Suppl 349], 1959

6. Bray GA, Davidson MB, Drenick EJ: Obesity: a serious symptom. Ann Intern Med 77:779-795, 1972

7. Bray GA, Gallagher TF Jr: Hypothalamic obesity in man: A study of eight patients and a review of the literature. Submitted

8. Bray GA: Measurement of subcutaneous fat cells from obese patients. Ann Intern Med 73:565-569, 1970

9. Bray GA, York D: Genetically transmitted obesity in rodents. Physiol Rev 51:598-646, 1971

10. Brecher G, Waxler SH: Obesity in albino mice due to single injections of gold thioglucose. Proc Soc Exp Biol Med 70:498-501, 1949

11. Brooks CM, Lambert EF: A study of the effect of limitations of food intake and the method of feeding on the rate of weight gain during hypothalamic obesity in the albino rat. Am J Physiol 147:695-707, 1946

12. Bullen BA, Reed RB, Mayer J: Physical activity of obese and nonobese adolescent girls appraised by motion picture sampling. Am J Clin Nutr 14:211-223, 1964

13. Chirico AM, Stunkard AJ: Physical activity and human obesity. N Engl J Med 263:935-940, 1960

14. Cohn C, Joseph D, Bell L, Allweiss MD: Studies on the effects of feeding frequency and dietary composition on fat deposition. Ann NY Acad Sci 131:507-518, 1965

15. Epstein AN, Teitelbaum P: Specific loss of the hypoglycemic control

of feeding in recovered lateral rats. Am J Physiol 213:1159-1167, 1967

16. Fabry P, Tepperman J: Meal frequency—a possible factor in human pathology. Am J Clin Nutr 23:1059-1068, 1970

17. Frohlich A: Ein Fall von Tumor der Hypophysis cerebri ohne Akromegale. Wien Klin Rund 15:883-886, 1901.

18. Frohman LA, Bernardis LL, Schnatz JD, Burck L: Plasma insulin and triglyceride levels after hypothalamus lesions in weanling rats. Am J Physiol 216:1496-1501, 1969.

19. Goldman JK, Schnatz JD, Bernardis LL, Frohman LA: Adipose tissue metabolism of weanling rats after destruction of ventromedial hypothalamic nuclei: Effect of hypophysectomy and growth hormone. Metabolism 19:995-1005, 1970

20. Goldman JK, Schnatz JD, Bernardis LL, Frohman LA: Effects of ventromedial hypothalamic destruction in rats with preexisting streptozotocin-induced diabetes. Metabolism 21:132-136, 1972

21. Goldzieher ZW, Green JA: The polycystic ovary. I. Clinical and histologic features. J Clin Endocrinol Metab 22:325-338, 1962

22. Haessler HA, Crawford JD: Fatty acid composition and metabolic activity of depot fat in experimental obesity. Am J Physiol 213:244-261, 1967

23. Hales CN, Kennedy GC: Plasma glucose, nonesterified fatty acids and insulin concentrations in hypothalamic-hyperphagic rats. Biochem J 90:620-624, 1964

24. Hall BD, Smith DW: Prader-Willi syndrome. J Pediatr 81:286-293, 1972

25. Henschen F: Morgagnis Syndrome: Hyperostosis Frontalis Interna, Virilismus, Obesitas. Edinburgh, Oliver and Boyd, 1949

26. Hirsch J, Gallian E: Methods for the determination of adipose cell size in man and animals. J Lipid Res 9:110-119, 1968

27. Hirsch J, Han P: Cellularity of rat adipose tissue: Effects of growth, starvation and obesity. J Lipid Res 10:77-82, 1969

28. Hirsch J, Knittle JL: Cellularity of obese and nonobese human adipose tissue. Fed Proc 29:1516-1521, 1970

29. Hoebel BG, Teitelbaum P: Weight regulation in normal and hypothalamic-hyperphagic rats. J Comp Physiol Psychol 61:189-193, 1966

30. Hollifield G: Glucocorticoid-induced obesity—a model and a challenge. Am J Clin Nutr 21:1471-1474, 1968

31. Ingle DJ: A simple means of producing obesity in the rat. Proc Soc Exp Biol Med 72:605-605, 1949

32. Jansen GR, Hutchison CF: Production of hypothalamic obesity by microsurgery. Am J Physiol 217:487-493, 1969

33. Jarlov E: The clinical types of abnormal obesity. Acta Med. Scand. (Suppl.) 42:1-70, 1932

34. Johnson PR, Hirsch J: The cellularity of adipose depots in 6 strains of genetically obese mice. J Lipid Res 13:2-11, 1972

35. Johnson PR, Zucker LM, Cruce JAF, Hirsch J: Cellularity of adipose depots in the genetically obese Zucker rat. J Lipid Res 12:706-714, 1971

36. Kavlie H, White TT: Pancreatic islet beta cell tumors and hyperplasia: Experience in 14 Seattle hospitals. Ann Surg 175:326-335, 1972

37. Kennedy GC: The role of depot fat in the hypothalamic control of food intake in the rat. Proc R Soc Lond [Biol] 140:578-592, 1953

38. Kennedy GC, Parker RA: The islets of Langerhans in rats with hypothalamic obesity. Lancet 2:981-982, 1963

39. Klein C, Ammann F: The syndrome of Laurence-Moon-Bardet-Biedl and allied diseases in Switzerland. J Neurol Sci 9:479-513, 1969

40. Lemmonier D: Effect of age, sex and site in the cellularity of the adipose tissue in mice and rats rendered obese by a high fat diet. J Clin Invest 51:2907-2915, 1972

41. Mabrey RE: Chordoma: A study of 150 cases. Am J Cancer 25:501-517, 1935

42. Mahler RJ, Szabo O: Amelioration of insulin resistance in obese mice. Am J Physiol 221:980-983, 1971

43. Mayer J: Genetic, traumatic and environmental factors in the etiology of obesity. Physiol Rev 33:472-508, 1953

44. Mayer J, Marshall NB, Vitale JJ, Christensen JH, Moshagekhi MB, Stare FJ: Exercise, food intake and body weight in normal rats and genetically obese adult mice. Am J Physiol 177:544-548, 1954

45. Noorden KV: Die Fettsucht. Nothnagel Spec Pathol Ther 7:1-156, 1900

46. Olney JW: Brain lesions, obesity and other disturbances in mice treated with monosodium glutamate. Science 64:719-721, 1969

47. Rutman MN, Lewis FS, Bloomer W: Metabolic investigations during the development of obesity in bipiperidyl mustard treated mice. Trans NY Acad Sci 30:244-255, 1967

48. Salans LB, Cushman SW, Weissman RE: Studies of human adipose tissue: Adipose cell size and number in nonobese and obese patients. J Clin Invest 52:929-941, 1973

49. Schemmel R, Mickelsen O, Gill JL: Dietary obesity in rats: Body weight and fat accretion· in seven strains of rats. J Nutr 100:1041-1048, 1970

50. Sjostrom L, Bjorntorp P, Vrana J: Microscopic fat cell size measurements on frozen-out adipose tissue in comparison with automatic determinations of osmium-fixed fat cells. J Lipid Res 12:521-530, 1971

51. Soffer LJ, Iannaccone A, Gabrilove JL: Cushing's syndrome. Am J Med 30:129-146, 1961

52. Stevenson JAF: Neural control of food and water intake, The Hypothalamus. Edited by W Haymaker, E Anderson, and WJH Nauter. Springfield, Ill, Charles C Thomas, 1969, pp. 524-621

53. Svolos DG: Craniopharyngiomas. Acta Chir Scand [Suppl 403] 1970

54. Teitelbaum P, Cheng MF, Rozin P: Stages of recovery and development of lateral hypothalamic control of food and water intake. Ann NY Acad Sci 157:849-860, 1969

55. Wade GN: Gonadal hormones and behavioral regulation of body weight. Physiol Behav 8:523-534, 1972

56. Yamamoto S, Mizutani T, Kaneuchi G: Obesity induced in mice injected intracerebrally with 4-nitro-quinoline 1-oxide or 4-hydroxy-aminoquinoline 1-oxide. Proc Soc Exp Biol Med 133:303-306, 1970

Disorders
of Lipid Metabolism

6

DAVID H. BLANKENHORN

Obesity, blood lipids, and vascular diseases are intimately related, and this review will cover some of the salient features of diagnosis and approaches to therapy. Elevations of blood lipid or lipoproteins can be conveniently classified into one of five types. Of these five, Type II and Type IV are clearly associated with vascular disease and have been called the high-risk hyperlipoproteinemias. Patients with Type IV abnormalities are often obese, and it is important to evaluate and treat the obesity. In Type II, obesity appears to be less important and less related to prevalence of coronary disease or degree of elevation of blood lipid. The differentiation of patients with Type IV, in whom weight reduction is critical in management, from patients with Type II, in whom weight control is less important, is one of the most useful contributions of current diagnostic tests.

The relationships of total cholesterol and triglyceride in the two "high-risk" hyperlipoproteinemias differ (Fig. 6-1). Plasma lipoprotein electrophoresis is one way to differentiate these two disorders. For this technique plasma is streaked with a pipet onto the filter paper strip in the area designated "origin." As electrophoresis proceeds, plasma proteins

Supported in part by USPHS Grants HL 14138 and RR 43.

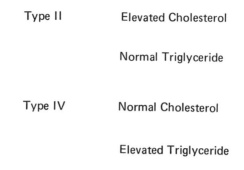

Type II	Elevated Cholesterol
	Normal Triglyceride
Type IV	Normal Cholesterol
	Elevated Triglyceride

Fig. 6-1. Cholesterol and triglycerides in the high-risk hyperlipoproteinemias.

migrate. The most rapidly moving component is albumin. Three of the components are important in the diagnosis of hyperlipoproteinemia and are identified on electrophoretic strips by staining with a fat-soluble dye such as oil red O and are thus termed lipoproteins (Fig. 6-2).

Alpha$_2$ lipoprotein, which migrates between alpha$_1$ lipoprotein and beta lipoprotein, is also frequently called prebeta lipoprotein. If ali-

Fig. 6-2. Scheme for phenotyping by electrophoresis to diagnose hyperlipoproteinemia. The two high-risk forms are differentiated by their mobilities.

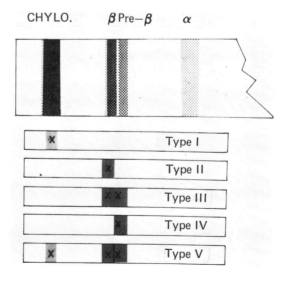

mentary fat particles or chylomicrons are present, these do not migrate, but remain at "origin" where plasma was placed on the paper strip.

Phenotyping by electrophoresis is used in diagnosing hyperlipoproteinemia (Fig. 6-3). In Type II hyperlipoproteinemia, beta lipoprotein is the principle component. In Type IV hyperlipoproteinemia, prebeta lipoprotein is the principle component which is elevated.

The clinical characteristics of patients with familial Type II hyperlipoproteinemia, which was formerly called familial xanthomatous hypercholesterolemia, are:

Cholesterol 300-500 mg/100 ml
Triglyceride under 300 mg/100 ml
Arcus, xanthelasma, tendon xanthomas
Premature coronary disease
Another hypercholesterolemic blood relative

The corneal arcus, which is frequently present, is different from the usual corneal arcus which most physicians are acquainted with. The common form of "senile" corneal arcus begins and is most prominent in the upper 180° of the cornea. The arcus of familial Type II hyperlipoproteinemia begins in the lower 180° of the cornea, usually at 4 o'clock or 7 o'clock. As the arcus of familial Type II enlarges, it can encircle the entire cornea, but if the patient has been observant, he will usually relate that when the arcus began, it was in the lower 180°.

Xanthelasmas are flat yellow lesions of the eyelid which usually begin on the inner canthus of the upper eyelid. As they grow, they usually involve both upper and lower eyelids. Not all xanthelasmas are signs of Type II hyperlipoproteinemia. They can occur when lipids are elevated in diabetes mellitus, myxedema, and biliary cirrhosis. In addition, there is a familial condition in which xanthelasmas occur without elevated blood cholesterol. In these families, the xanthelasmas usually occur in women at the time of the menopause.

Another characteristic lesion of Type II hyperlipoproteinemia is the tendinous xanthoma. It is rare to see tendon xanthomas as large as those now frequently shown in textbook illustrations. The vast majority of Type II patients with tendon xanthomas have small lesions on the extensor tendons of the hands or the Achilles tendons. Xanthomas on the hands are usually overlooked or confused with small exostoses. Tendon xanthomas can be distinguished from exostoses by any manuever which causes the tendon to move through the joint because xanthomas will move with the tendons whereas exostoses remain fixed in relation to the joint. Xanthomas of the Achilles tendon are best recognized by slight asymmetry of the tendon or a posterior bulging just above its implantation into the calcaneus. Achilles tendon xanthomas are most noticeable when the patient puts his weight on his feet, and they are frequently overlooked when the patient is examined lying with feet extended and tendons relaxed. If there is doubt as to whether these xanthomas are present, lateral x-ray films of the ankle will resolve the problem.

Nonfamilial Type II hyperlipoproteinemia is a less severe form, in which xanthomas are much less common and no family history is present. This type, formerly known as undifferentiated hypercholesterolemia, has the following characteristics:

Level in upper 10% of age group
Nondiabetic
Nonhypothyroid
Family history negative or unknown
Fasting LPEP variable, no chylomicrons, low VLDL, or prebeta lipoprotein

Abnormalities of the nonfamilial Type II respond more readily to therapy than the familial type. In treating either condition, it is desirable to lower the cholesterol content of diet and to increase the ratio of polyunsaturated to saturated fatty acids. To treat nonfamilial Type II, a diet in which cholesterol intake is less than 300 mg/day, with a 2:1 ratio of polyunsaturated fatty acid to saturated fatty acid, is adequate. Fat calories should comprise 40% of total calories.

Familial Type II hyperlipoproteinemia should be treated rigorously with reduction of cholesterol intake to less than 200 mg/day. The ratio of polyunsaturated fatty acid to saturated fatty acid should approach 3:1. Fat (calories as fat) should be reduced to approximately 30%. Weight loss is not an important means of altering cholesterol in either familial or nonfamilial Type II hyperlipoproteinemia. Obese patients with either of these conditions should, however, lose weight for the same reasons that obese people in general should lose weight. During periods of active weight loss, cholesterol levels may be lower, but no very noticeable or sustained change in blood lipids will occur.

Drug therapy for patients with Type II hyperlipoproteinemia includes resins which bind bile acids, such as cholestyramine or cholesterol. The dose of cholestyramine is 18-24 g/day. Another promising therapeutic regimen is the combination of oral neomycin sulfate, 1 g twice a day, and clofibrate (Atromid-S), 1 g twice a day.

The clinical picture of Type IV hyperlipoproteinemia is less definitive. It is one of the most common yet one of the most poorly defined hyperlipoproteinemias. It is quite common among patients with premature coronary disease—i.e., those whose first myocardial infarction occurred before the age of 50. In addition to elevated levels of triglyceride, many of these patients have abnormal glucose tolerance curves. Thus, Type IV hyperlipoproteinemia may also be intimately related to adult-onset diabetes mellitus.

Another characteristic of Type IV hyperlipoproteinemia is that it is exacerbated by a high carbohydrate diet. In fact, Type IV hyperlipoproteinemia was discovered when it was found that certain patients with elevated triglycerides did not respond to a low-fat diet with a fall in triglycerides, but instead showed a marked increase. This observation led to reevaluation of the earlier view that alimentary triglycerides (fats) were the major source of elevated blood triglycerides in man. A typical response to a high carbohydrate diet is shown in Figure 6-6. A 42-year-old woman with coronary disease and Type IV hyperlipoproteinemia was given a liquid formula diet which provided 87% of the calories as carbohydrate and approximately 1% of the calories as fat. A brisk rise in triglyceride occurred. Most patients with Type IV hyperlipoproteinemia show such a rise between the second and fifth days on a high carbohydrate diet. Less rigorous dietary tests can also elicit this response, but the triglycerides rise more slowly and to a lesser extent.

The clinical characteristics of patients with Type IV hyperlipoproteinemia may be summarized as follows:

Usually no family history or physical findings
Triglycerides 200-800 mg/100 ml, transported as prebeta lipoproteins
Triglycerides labile and fall with weight loss
Triglycerides rise on high carbohydrate diet
Cholesterol usually normal

Weight reduction is one of the most effective treatments for patients with Type IV hyperlipoproteinemia. Most therapeutic programs should

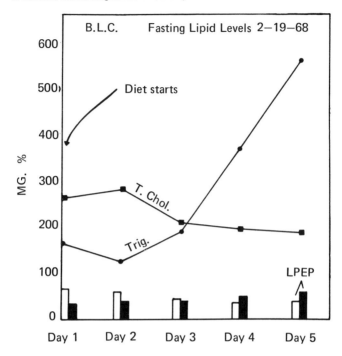

Fig. 6-3. Effects of high carbohydrate diet in 42-year-old woman with coronary disease and Type IV hyperlipoproteinemia. Note sharp rise in triglycerides and decline and leveling off of cholesterol.

begin here because the vast majority of adults with Type IV hyperlipopro-teinemia are overweight. In my experience, patients with Type IV hyperlipoproteinemia are approximately 25-40 lb above ideal body weight. A prompt fall in plasma triglyceride occurs as soon as weight reduction begins and appears to be sustained as long as weight reduction is maintained. At the same time, glucose tolerance shows marked improve-ment, suggesting once again the close relationship between Type IV hyperlipoproteinemia and adult-onset diabetes mellitus.

The mechanism by which weight reduction improves Type IV hyper-lipoproteinemia is not clearly understood. The major portion of the elevated triglyceride in this condition is transported by the alpha$_2$ or prebeta lipoprotein. It is also known that the fatty acid part of the triglycerides in prebeta lipoproteins is derived from fatty acids liberated from storage depots in fat cells. During periods of starvation, free fatty acids are liberated from depot fat. Most of these free fatty acids are metabolized by tissues, such as skeletal muscle and heart, and provide one of the major sources of energy in fasting individuals. Those free fatty acids that are not used to meet the energy requirements of working tissue are removed from blood by the liver and reformed into triglyceride. This triglyceride, the so-called endogenous triglyceride is transported in plasma as prebeta or alpha$_2$ lipoprotein. It is not presently known whether the elevation of prebeta lipoprotein is caused by too rapid entry of prebeta lipoprotein into blood or too sluggish removal from blood. Despite this lack of information, it seems clear that reduction of the formation of endogenous triglyceride will eventually cause a fall in the circulating level of prebeta lipoproteins. Reduction in prebeta lipoprotein can be accomplished by weight reduction because weight reduction lowers the amount of free fatty acid available to the liver for formation of endogenous triglyceride. During the acute period of weight loss, the availability of free fatty acids to the liver is reduced because free fatty acids are metabolized to make up caloric deficits. When body weight is stabilized at a lower level, free fatty acid mobilization is reduced. This occurs because the relative change in body composition means less depot fat is available to provide free fatty acids and relatively more skeletal muscle is available to metabolize these free fatty acids. Thus, formation of endogenous prebeta lipoproteins is reduced.

REFERENCES

1. Frederickson DS, Levy RI, Lees RS: Fat transport in lipoproteins. An integrated approach to mechanisms and disorders. N Engl J Med 276:32-44, 94-103, 148-156, 215-226, 273-281, 1967
2. Levy RI, Fredrickson DS, Shulman R, Bilheimer DW, Breslow JL, Stone NJ, Lux SE, Sloan HR, Krauss RM, Herbert PN: Dietary and drug treatment of primary hyperlipoproteinemia. Ann Intern Med 77:267-294, 1972

The Ills of the Obese

7

D. W. PETIT

The obese tend to be a sickly lot—the more obese, the more sickly. Any physician who has spent time caring for these patients can attest to this. This belief comes from general impressions and a sort of common-sense appraisal of the abrasive effects of time and society on the obese. It is with this bias and prejudice that the ills of the obese are to be discussed. For those who wish a refreshing view of an opposite bias, there is a delightful article by G. V. Mann (14) entitled "Obesity, the Nutritional Spook."

Any discussion of illness and obesity must deal with concepts of cause and effect. At this time there is no consensus regarding the etiology of obesity. Moreover, at this time there is no incontrovertible evidence that weight loss cures the ills of the obese. Obesity is a sociophysical diagnosis, a combination of what the mirror says, what tables of height and weight say, and what the biochemist says. There is a good discussion of various techniques for evaluating obesity, ranging from estimates of cadaver fat, to the simple use of observation, in the publication "Obesity and Health" (19). The ills of the obese will be catalogued in four areas, no one of which should be considered independent of the others. These four are:

Manifest disease
Biochemical and metabolic abnormalities

Social interactions
Costs and hazards of therapy

The role of weight reduction in lessening the ills of the obese can best be appraised by a willingness to examine each of these four areas for each obese person and then proceed with therapy after that. The question must be posed of whether there are varying degrees of risk faced by people with different forms of obesity. Can these risk factors be measured? Should our efforts at relieving the ills of the obese be concentrated on such people rather than on the total population of the obese? Some attempt will be made in the four areas mentioned above to identify such high-risk situations.

MANIFEST DISEASE

Life shortening high-risk disease (1, 11, 12, 16, 17, 23)
    Hypertension
    Diabetes mellitus
    Sudden death predisposition
    Respiratory insufficiency
    Toxemia of pregnancy
    Thromboembolic disease
    Congestive heart failure
Moderate to severe morbidity (6, 19, 20)
    Gallstones
    Osteoarthritis
    Varices
    Hernias
    Menstrual disturbances
    Depression
    Anxiety
    Anesthetic risk
Discomfiture and impaired life style
    Dermatitis
    Flat feet
    Impaired agility
    Heat intolerance

As one moves along the scale from life threatening to discomfiture, one has the impression that the ills faced by the obese are more certainly helped by weight reduction as one gets into the less serious aspects of their illness. It is in precisely the highest risk group that the greatest uncertainty exists regarding the help that may be offered. This is particularly the case with the moderately obese. The hugely obese patient is more certainly benefited by efforts at weight reduction. At least this would seem to be true in short-term studies. (3, 19) Quantitation of the hazards faced by the obese is meager. One has the impression that there is a great gap in our knowledge concerning the exact measurement of illness among the obese. Keys (12), in particular protests the lumping of all obese people together as prone to develop coronary artery disease.

BIOCHEMICAL-METABOLIC ABNORMALITIES (2, 21)

May be affected favorably by weight loss (10, 15, 21, 22)
Hyperlipidemia
Hypercholesterolemia
Hyperinsulinemia
Insulin resistance
Decreased glucose tolerance
Increased cortisol secretion
Size of fat cells

Probably unaffected by weight loss
Numbers of fat cells
Any genetic predisposition to obesity

The work of Sims *et al.* (21) has established the inducibility and reversibility of most of the above-mentioned abnormalities. Similarly, the work of Stern *et al.* (22) and others has shown the inability to affect the number of fat cells by simple weight loss. Brook (4) has suggested that there may be a sensitive period in adipose cell replication lasting from the 30th week of gestation through the 52nd postpartum week, during which time the number of fat cells may be subject to regulation by food intake.

The first two categories of ills—namely, manifest disease and biochemical-metabolic abnormalities—are, at this time, still very poorly quantitated, but they do begin to establish a way by which there might be some profile in the examination of every obese person that would identify those who are at high risk. Such identification would temper the therapeutic program to be undertaken. There are, however, two other categories of problems that beset the obese that cannot be overlooked.

SOCIAL INTERACTIONS

The following problems are each of increasing severity as the degree of obesity increases:

Impaired job opportunities
Impaired educational opportunities
Larger percent of income necessary for clothes and food
Impaired quality of medical care
Increased susceptibility to advertising and general allures of food industry (18)
Problems with heterosexual relationships
Problems of self-identification in the raising of obese children. (9)

It is frequently overlooked that there are definite limitations to the weight level that a person may have in order to be employed. Felton (7, 8) in discussing aspects of this sort in Los Angeles County, estimated that this was a particular problem faced by minority groups from deprived areas in the county. Problems of the cost of living are often disregarded or literally swept under the rug. Anyone who has worked with the severely obese knows that the majority of these patients wish to have extra funds for diet, while those who pay from public funds for such diets are inclined to scoff. Calories are not free, but some are cheaper than others. The cost of 3500-4000 Cal/day, however, is going to be greater than 2000/day, at any level of living. (13) The poor who are obese have just that much less money available as disposable income than the poor who are lean.

Similarly, one of the factors that can unconsciously delay weight reduction is the cost of changing the size of clothing. The problems of quality of medical care faced by the obese vary in relationship to the magnitude of their problem. These factors range from the sheer mechanical problems associated with all medical procedures to the negative attitudes held by many physicians toward the obese. Problems of agility are self-evident. An interesting concept of this was discussed in an article by Wilmore and Pruitt (24), entitled "Fat Boys Get Burned," in which they indicated the increased chance for that particular type of trauma among the obese as opposed to the nonobese.

The final category of problems facing the obese deals with weight loss.

COSTS AND HAZARDS OF WEIGHT REDUCTION THERAPY

Hazards of drugs
Hazards of surgery
Dollar costs of therapy
Hazards of unsupervised therapy
Hazards of psychotherapy and counseling
Hazards of rapid weight loss
    Gouty attacks
    Fatty change in the liver
    Orthostatic hypotension and syncope
    Loss of lean body mass

Edison (5) has described well the problems associated with the amphetamines. The difficulties associated with rapid weight loss, whether it comes from starvation or bypass surgery, are discussed in some detail by Bray *et al.* (3).

The obese deserve careful study—the more obese, the more detailed the study should be. Weight loss may be helpful to some and the potential must be weighed against the hazards and costs of therapy. If the evidence becomes more conclusive regarding the harmful effects of moderate, as well as severe obesity, and if there comes stronger evidence of the value of weight loss, it will be necessary to enlist the aid of the food industry in orienting the selling practices of food (13). The hazards faced by the obese must be considered as a mosaic of ills. It is important to sort out among the obese those whom weight loss can benefit from those who may be far more affected by therapy than by their obesity. There is little to be gained in a normotensive, normocholesterolemic, normolipemic, nondiabetic obese adult, who is functioning well in his society by arousing anxieties concerning his weight. On the other hand, a hypertensive obese person, with hyperlipemia and diabetes, who is smoking a pack of cigarettes per day, needs all the aid that can be given to alter his life style. What is needed at this time is the development of a technique for detecting the high risk obese individuals and concentrating our efforts upon them.

REFERENCES

1. Alexander JK: Cardiovascular effects of obesity. Medical Counterpoint, September 1970, pp. 15-28

2. Bortz WM: Metabolic consequences of obesity. Ann Inter Med 71:833-843, 1969

3. Bray G: Obesity: A serious symptom. Ann Intern Med 77:779-796, 1972

4. Brook CGD: Evidence for a sensitive period in adipose-cell replication in man. Lancet 2:624-627, 1972

5. Edison GR: Amphetamines: A dangerous illusion. Ann Intern Med 74:605-610, 1971

6. Feinberg GL: Obesity: Class IV anesthesia risk NY State J Med 71:2200-2201, 1971

7. Felton JS: Occupational health. JAMA 217:56-60, 1971

8. Felton JS: Personal comments

9. Garell DC: The obese person as an adolescent. Calif Med 000:368-371, 1967

10. Gates RJ: Return to normal of blood-glucose, plasma-insulin and weight gain in New Zealand obese mice after implantation of islets of langerhans. Lancet 2:567-570, 1972

11. Kannel WB: Relations of body weight to development of coronary heart disease—the Framingham study. Circulation 35:735-744, 1967

12. Keys A: Coronary heart disease: Overweight and obesity as risk factors. Ann Intern Med 77:15-27, 1972

13. Lowe CU: Nutrition and national goals. Med Opin Rev 000:104-113, 1968

14. Mann GV: Obesity, the nutritional spook. Am J Public Health 61:1491-1498, 1971

15. Mayer J: Some aspects of the problem of regulation of food intake and obesity. N Engl J Med 274:610-616, 662-673, 722-731, 1966

16. Mortality Among Overweight Men. Statistical Bull., Metropolitan Life Ins. Co. 41:6-11, 1960

17. Mortality Among Overweight Women. Statistical Bull., Metropolitan Life Ins. Co. 41:2-5, 1960

18. Nisbett RE: Taste, depreciation, and weight determination of eating behavior. Pers Soc Psychol 10:107-116, 1968

19. Obesity and Health. USPHS, HEW, U.S. Government Printing Office, 1966

20. Rimm AA: Disease and obesity in 73,532 women. Obesity Bariatr Med 1:77-84, 1972

21. Sims EAH: Inducible metabolic abnormalities during development of obesity. Annu Rev Med 22:235-251, 1971

22. Stern JS: Adipose-cell size and immuno-reactive insulin levels in obese and normal weight adults. Lancet 2:948-950, 1972

23. Walsh RE: Upper airway obstruction in obese patients with sleep disturbance and somnolency. Ann Intern Med 76:185-182, 1972

24. Wilmore DW, Pruitt BA: Fat boys get burned. Lancet 2:631-632, 1972

NEWER **III**
APPROACHES
TO THE TREATMENT
OF OBESITY

Effects of Diet and Exercise in the Treatment of Obesity

8

GRANT GWINUP

The decision to treat an obese patient depends on several considerations: (1) the degree of fatness in relation to the ideal levels of body weight for the individual; (2) motivation to lose weight and (3) the presence of diseases whose course is complicated by obesity. For most adolescents in this society, body fat content ranges from 15% to 23%, being several percentage points higher in females than in males, particularly after puberty. A body-fat content of 5% would provide an energy reserve sufficient for 1-2 weeks without food. Larger stores, which most of us have, provide substantially greater quantities of energy fuel and are analogous to an automobile towing a 500-gallon fuel tank behind it rather than stopping for fuel as needed every 200-300 miles. The relationship of body fat to age compounds our interpretation of "ideal" percent of body fat. All longitudinal studies which have examined this question find that the percentage of fat in both males and females increases with age (Fig, 8-1). This increase is usually accompanied by a decrease in lean body mass

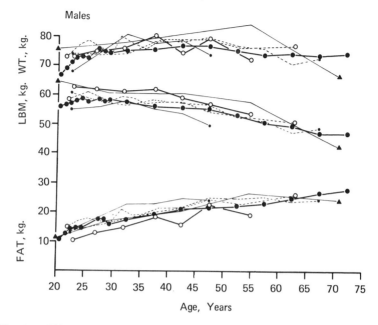

Fig. 8-1. Effects of age on body composition in several studies. Body weight increased slightly with age. Body fat rose more and lean body mass (*LBM*) declined. (Forbes GB, Reina JC: Adult lean body mass declines with age: some longitudinal observations. Metabolism 19:653-663, 1970)

and a small increase in total body weight. Thus, for males, body fat can rise from 18% to 20% at age 20, to 35% by age 60, wtih little change in body weight and a corresponding decrease in lean body mass (7). It would seem desirable to maintain body fat content in ranges no higher than 20-25% for men, and 25-30% for women.

Since the stores of body fat in the adipose tissue depots represent stores of energy, considerable attention has been paid to the processes which regulate this quantity of stored energy. Current evidence suggests that some component of the total amount of body fat serves as a signal to regulate the ingestion and/or expenditure of energy. Two kinds of evidence would support this contention. The first is provided by studies in which parts of the body fat are removed by surgically amputating depots of adipose tissue. When this occurs, experimental animals will regain body fat in other depots until their total content of fat has returned to its original level (12).

Similarly, in experimental animals which have been attached to one another so that there is a slow but constant cross-circulation from one to the other, food regulation can be disturbed by making one animal develop a form of experimental obesity by injury of the hypothalamus (for detailed discussions, see Chapter 5). When this happens, the animal with the lesion becomes fat, but the attached animal without the lesion decreases its total body fat content (10). Thus, the animal with the intact central nervous system senses some factor from the animal that is becoming obese which tells the lean animal to eat less and correspondingly become less fat. These two lines of evidence argue that something in the total body fat serves to help regulate it at a present level. Treatment of obesity involves efforts to alter total body fat. If the body has mechanisms for controlling body fat at some set level, such therapeutic attempts may be very difficult to accomplish at best.

DIETARY TREATMENT

The general approaches to the problem of weight reduction take two forms. The first involves efforts to decrease total caloric intake, and the second involves ways of increasing caloric expenditure primarily through exercise (3). There are three considerations in the use of diet for obesity: (1) the total caloric needs of a patient and the degree of caloric restriction which is desired; (2) the distribution of these calories between carbohydrate, protein, and fat to provide a balanced diet; and (3) the frequency with which food is eaten. Over the past 70 years, a voluminous amount of information has accumulated concerning human metabolic requirements. The evidence indicates that caloric needs can be divided into two components. One is the so-called basal metabolic requirements (BMR— basal metabolic rate)—*i.e.,* those calories used for digestion of food, for maintenance of normal body tissues, and for brain function, etc. Basal metabolic needs are slightly lower for women than for men, but in general are approximately 1000 Cal/sqm of surface area per day. The surface area or amount of external surface varies with height and weight. A 150-lb man standing 5 ft 10 in. tall has 1.7 sqm of surface area.

In addition to the basal metabolic needs, there are the needs for physical activity. For the average American 15-20 years, this is approximately 60% more than the basal metabolic rate. The calories required for physical activity decline gradually to approximately 40% of the basal metabolic rate for people over 60 years of age. Thus, a woman aged 15-19 years, standing 5 ft tall and weighing 100 lb, would require approximately 2000 Cal for normal levels of activity. For a woman 6 ft tall, weighing 145 lb, this would rise to 2800 Cal. Over the ensuing years to age 60, these figures would fall to approximately 1500 Cal for a woman 5 ft tall and just over 2000 Cal for a woman 6 ft tall.

For men, the figures are somewhat higher. Men aged 15-19 years who are 5 ft tall require 2600 Cal and those 6 ft tall, 3400 Cal. The corresponding figures for men aged 60-69 are 1700 and 2200 Cal. Thus, an accurate assessment of total caloric requirement involves knowledge of both the basal caloric requirement, which varies with age and size of the individual, and the calories needed for physical activity. Clearly, the caloric intake that will suffice to keep people of the same height at constant weight will vary widely largely because of the differences in the numbers of calories expended by varying degrees of activity.

After the assessment of total caloric requirement, the next goal is to provide a reasonable caloric deficit. By caloric deficit, I mean the difference between calories required to maintain weight and the actual calories in the prescribed diet. If a caloric deficit of 1000 Cal is prescribed and maintained, a loss of 7000 Cal will be incurred during 1 wk of this regime. Since each pound of fatty tissue contains approximately 3500 Cal, this means that with a 1000-Cal deficit each day, 2 lb of fatty tissue will be consumed each week to provide for the extra calories for metabolism and activity (4). In patients with large caloric requirements, a severe degree of caloric restriction may be unacceptable, and it is usually best to provide a calorie deficit that is no more than 500-1500 Cal/day. Occasionally, however, exceptions to these limits will be necessary.

With adherence to any diet, two phases of weight loss are observed. The first is the initial rapid phase which reflects in large part the loss of fluids as the body adjusts to utilizing its stored fatty depots. After some days, this fluid is depleted and subsequent weight loss reflects primarily losses of weight by catabolism of fat (15). Since this occurs at a slower rate than the weight loss by excreting fluid, most patients become distressed with the slowness of progress after the first 2-3 wk. A second component of this frustration is the tendency of some individuals to adapt to caloric restriction by decreasing their caloric expenditure (2) (Fig. 8-2). If this happens, the prescribed diet produces a smaller loss of weight than

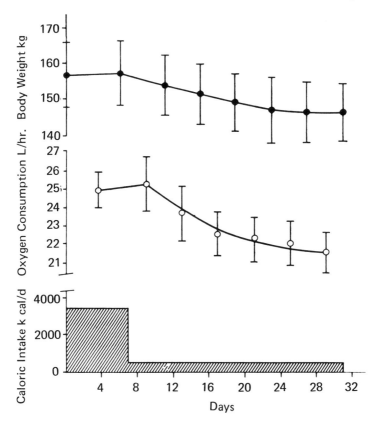

Fig. 8-2. Effect of caloric restriction on body weight and oxygen consumption. When caloric intake was decreased from 3600 to 450 kCal/day, oxygen consumption declined and the rate of weight loss which was initially rapid slowed. (Bray GA: Effect of caloric restriction on energy expenditure in obese patients. Lancet 2:397-398, 1968)

anticipated, leading to even greater frustration on the part of the patient. In carefully controlled situations, however, it is possible, with knowledge of basal metabolic requirements and energy expenditure, to predict with reasonable accuracy the rates of weight loss over extended periods of time.

New diets are frequently appearing in the popular magazines and in book form. This suggests that no one of them is ideal, since if it were, we would not see a need for continuing resurgence of new diets. One of the frequently recurring diets is the low-carbohydrate, high-fat diet propounded intermittently since the time of Banting nearly 100 years ago (1). The question that this diet raises is whether a diet imbalanced in one or another of its major nutrients is more beneficial in producing weight loss than a diet which is reasonably balanced. Two groups of workers have provided discrepant data on this question. In the careful studies of Kinsell *et al.* (11) and by Pilkington *et al.* (16), the answer would appear to be no. For these studies, patients were hospitalized and the fraction of calories provided as fat, carbohydrate, and proteins was varied over a wide range. After the initial phase of weight loss due to the excretion of water, these investigators found that variation in the distribution of calories between carbohydrates, fat, and protein seemed to have no influence on the rate at which weight was lost.

Recent studies by Young *et al.* (17) has suggested, on the other hand, that a very low carbohydrate diet may indeed increase the rate at which body fat is catabolized. Their studies, on a small number of college students, require confirmation before they can be fully accepted. However, they suggest that a carbohydrate content of less than 50 g/day in the diet is sufficient to cause increased rates of weight loss compared to 60-104 g of carbohydrate in a diet with the same total number of calories. Thus, the question of the value of a low carbohydrate diet and its effectiveness in weight loss is still unresolved (19).

The frequency with which food is ingested may also be important in a weight control program. Several studies suggest that the frequency with which food is eaten does not change the rate of weight loss. We found between one feeding and nine feedings a day did not influence the quantity of weight loss over a given period of time (9). However, we and others have shown in college males, the frequency of feedings did have profound influence on carbohydrate tolerance and on the level of cholesterol (9, 18). When normal college subjects were fed a weight-maintenance or a weight-reduction diet in one meal, they showed impairment of their glucose tolerance curves and higher levels of plasma cholesterol compared to the same diet fed in three or six equal feedings. (Table 8-1) This data would suggest that it is wise to eat three or more meals per day if for no other reason than that this regime seems to lower plasma cholesterol significantly and leads to some improvement in glucose tolerance.

Table 8-1 Frequency of Feeding on Serum Lipids

No. of Meals	No. Subjects	Serum Cholesterol	Serum Triglyceride
		mg/100 ml	mg/100 ml
6	8	259.5 ± 58.3	123.6 ± 46.0
3	6	266.5 ± 30.0 ⎫ P<.001	122.8 ± 53.5 ⎫ P<.05
1	8	305.9 ± 45.6 ⎭	166.8 ± 54.7 ⎭

Adapted from Young, C. M. *et al.* J. Am. Diet. Assoc. 59:478, 1971.

PHYSICAL EXERCISE

Effects of exercise on weight loss are clear. In persons who voluntarily increase their energy expenditure without a corresponding increase in food intake, extra weight is lost. The relationship between food intake and energy expenditure in exercise has been studied in both experimental and clinical states. In the experimental animal, the food intake and duration of exercise are closely related. If experimental animals are exercised between 1 and 5 hours per day, there is an increase in food intake which corresponds with the duration of exercise; body weight remains constant (13) (Fig. 8-3). When exercise is greater than 6 hours per day, food intake levels off and then declines and body weight falls.

Of greater interest for this sedentary society in which we live are the studies on restriction in activity. As activity is reduced below 1 hour per day in animals, food intake no longer falls but levels off and then actually rises, followed by an increase in body weight. Studies in India in a large industrial plant suggest that a similar relationship between degrees of activity and food intake may be present in humans (14). At low levels of energy expenditure—*i.e.,* the executive and administrative personnel—body weight and food intake were higher than in the intermediate levels of workers. Other data also indicate the relative inactivity of obese subjects, whether adolescent or adult. These data were obtained by Chirico and Stunkard (6) using pedometers and by Bullen *et al.* (5) from time-lapse motion picture studies. In both instances, it appeared that the obese subjects, whether adolescents in a summer camp or working adults, were less active in their obese state than were the nonobese controls. Thus, the obese are inactive, and inactivity may increase food intake. These facts

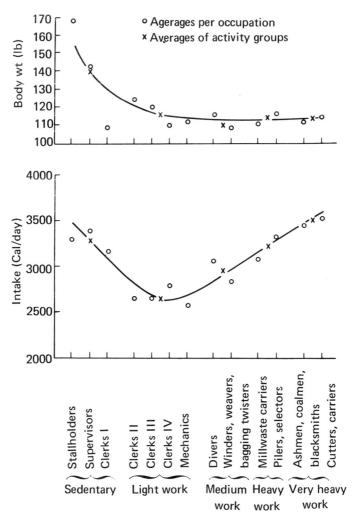

Fig. 8-3. Food intake and body weight related to occupational classification. Note that with sedentary occupations food intake and body weight both increased. (Mayer J, Roy P, Nitra RP: Relation between caloric intake, body weight and physical work. Am J Clin Nutr 4:169-175, 1956)

provide strong arguments of the need for some form of physical activity as part of any weight-reducing program.

Two kinds of physical activities are available (3): those which involve aerobic expenditure of energy, such as bicycling, swimming, or running; and those which are primarily anaerobic such as calisthenics, weight lifting, etc. There is evidence to suggest that the optimal effects on the cardiovascular system and probably the optimal state for lowering food intake and body weight can be achieved by relatively constant but low levels of aerobic activities. The amount of activity must be such as to raise the pulse rate somewhat at each session of activity and must be continued for a considerable length of time.

The importance of the rate at which various activities are undertaken has been pointed out in studies of Givoni and Goldman (8). If walking on a treadmill at constant rate but with increasing degree of slope is compared with walking up a constant slope but an increasing speed rate, there is a greater expenditure of energy by walking faster as compared to walking up a steeper slope. It is thought that the underlying mechanisms for this difference in effect of rate of walking are related to the inefficiency of moving the legs more rapidly as compared to the work accomplished by walking up an increasing grade. For these reasons, it seems highly important to undertake walking or any other activity at a sufficiently rapid rate to provide the beneficial effects to the cardiovascular system of increasing pulse rate and cardiac output, as well as providing maximum caloric utilization by performing work at a comfortable yet rapid pace.

REFERENCES

1. Banting W: Letter on corpulence addressed to the Public. Ed. 2, London, Harrison, 1863
2. Bray GA: Effect of caloric restriction on energy expenditure in obese patients. Lancet 2:397-398, 1969
3. Bray GA: Clinical management of the obese adult. Postgrad Med 51:125-130, 1972
4. Bortz WM: Predictability of weight loss. JAMA 204:101-105, 1968
5. Bullen BA, Reed RB, Mayer J: Physical activity of obese and nonobese adolescent girls appraised by motion picture sampling. Am J Clin Nutr 14:211-223, 1964

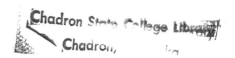

6. Chirico AM, Stunkard AJ: Physical activity and human obesity. N Engl J Med 263:935, 1960

7. Forbes GB, Reina JC: Adult lean body mass declines with age: some longitudinal observations. Metabolism 19:653-663, 1970

8. Givoni B, Goldman RF: Predicting metabolic energy cost. J Appl Physiol 30:429-433, 1971

9. Gwinup G, Byron RC, Roush WH, Kruger FA, Hamwi GJ: Effect of nibbling versus gorging on serum lipids in man. Am J Clin Nutr 13:209-213, 1963

10. Harvey GR: Physiological mechanisms in the regulation of energy balance. Symposium on Anorexia Nervosa & Obesity. The Royal College of Physicians of Edinburgh, Great Britain, 1973

11. Kinsell LW, Gunning B, Michaels GP, Richardson J, Cox SE, Lennon C: Calories do count. Metabolism 13:195-204, 1964

12. Liebelt RA, Ichinoe S, Nicholson N: Regulatory influences of adipose tissue on food intake and body weight. Ann NY Acad Sci 131:559-582, 1965

13. Mayer J, Marshall NB, Vitale JJ, Christensen JH, Mashayekhi MB, Sture FJ: Exercise, food intake and body weight in normal rats and genetically obese adult rats. Am J Physiol 177:544-548, 1954

14. Mayer J, Roy P, Mitra RP: Relation between caloric intake, body weight and physical work. Am J Clin Nutr 4:169-175, 1956.

15. Passmore R, Strong JA, Ritchie FJ: The chemical composition of the tissue lost by obese patients on a reducing regimen. Br J Nutr 12:113-121, 1968

16. Pilkington TRE, Gainsborough H, Rosenoer VM, Carey M: Diet and weight reduction in the obese. Lancet 1:856-858, 1960

17. Young CM, Scanlan SS, Im HS, Lutwak L: Effect on body composition and other parameters in obese young men of carbohydrate level of reduction diet. Am J Clin Nutr 24:290-296, 1971

18. Young CM, Scanlan SS, Topping CM, Simko V, Lutwak L: Frequency of feeding, weight reduction, and body composition. J Am Diet Assoc 59:466-472, 1971

19. Yudkin J: This Slimming Business. Penguin Handbooks. 3rd edition, 1971

New Treatments for Obesity: Behavior Modification

9

ALBERT STUNKARD

The treatment which I will discuss is directed toward the mildly or moderately obese and represents a significant advance in our approach to this disorder. As is well known, the usual results of outpatient treatment for obesity are extremely bad. Most obese patients won't even come for treatment. Those who do come often drop out. The ones who don't drop out, don't lose much weight. Finally, those who do lose weight usually regain it.

To quantify this dismal tale, we surveyed the medical literature and summarized the results of treatment for obesity. We took all the reports in a 10-year period and calculated what percentage of patients who entered treatment lost significant amounts of weight. There was a remarkable degree of unanimity in these results. No more than 25% of the patients lost as much as 20 lb and no more than 5% lost as much as 40 lb (8). That is not a very good record.

A new era in the treatment of obesity began in 1967 with the publication of a short paper, by a social worker named Richard Stuart, in a small psychology journal (5). Stuart's patients lost far more weight than any other group of obese patients treated on an outpatient basis (Fig. 9-1). As the results are examined, one should bear in mind that, in general, no more than 25% of obese persons lose 20 lb, and no more than 5% lose 40 lb.

The patients were treated by Stuart with a method known as behavior modification, over a period of 1 year. All lost more than 20 lb, 6 lost more than 30 lb, and 3 lost over 40 lb. These results are the best ever reported for outpatient treatment of obesity, and they constitute a landmark in our understanding of this disorder. Even the absence of a control group does not vitiate their significance. These remarkable results were achieved by a man who had had no previous experience in the treatment of obesity. And they were achieved with relatively small expenditures of time. Stuart saw his patients individually for half-hour visits three times a week for a month. After those 12 visits, he saw them infrequently for the next year. The total number of sessions was no more than 41 and as few as 16.

The basis for this treatment program had been laid down some years ago by Charles Ferster, one of the foremost students of B.F. Skinner. Ferster *et al.* (1) devised a very extensive program, with many sophisticated aspects. However, this program attracted little attention at the time, partly because Ferster did not report the results of his treatment, and partly because those who inquired about them learned that they were not very good. But Ferster had the idea and Stuart made it work.

Stuart's work initiated an explosion of research into the applications of behavior modification to the treatment of obesity. At least 10 papers on the topic have appeared in the 6 years since Stuart's paper, and another 10 studies have not yet been reported. It seems particularly important that physicians know of these developments in behavior modification, for this field has grown up largely outside of medical purview and, at times, in the face of medical opposition. The extent of the leadership exercised by psychologists and social workers is nowhere better illustrated than in the "medical" problem of obesity: Physicians participated in only one of the studies that I will describe.

The first study to follow Stuart's was carried out by Mary Harris, who was then working at Stanford (3). Dr. Harris's study, along with all of the other studies which I will describe, differed from Stuart's in two respects:

(1) Patients were treated in groups; and (2) the weight losses of groups treated by behavior modification were compared to the weight losses of control groups (Fig. 9-2).

The subjects were not really very obese. They were Stanford students who started with an average weight of 170 lb and lost an average of 8 pounds during 2.5 months of treatment. They continued to lose weight in the follow-up period. To Dr. Harris's good fortune, the control group gained weight, and her results were accordingly very highly significant from the statistical point of view ($p < 0.001$).

There was a flaw in Dr. Harris's study, however, and she called attention to it. Her control group did not receive treatment when the behavior modification group did, although they were told that they would be put on a waiting list for treatment. Now the use of a deferred-treatment control group raises a serious problem. For when people coming for treatment do not receive it, this is not a neutral event. In fact, it could be a discouraging event, and it may quite possibly have been the reason the control group gained weight.

Psychotherapy research needs, in addition to a no-treatment or deferred-treatment control group, a placebo control group. Until a short time ago, however, there had never been any placebo controls in psychotherapy research. Two graduate students at the University of Illinois took this important step.

The first study was carried out by Janet Wollersheim (9), who established four different experimental conditions: (1) focal behavior modification, 20 patients; (2) nonspecific therapy, 20 patients; (3) social pressure, 20 patients; (4) deferred-treatment control, 19 patients.

Her study thus contained three treatment conditions (1, 2, and 3) and three control conditions (2, 3, and 4). Four therapists treated groups of five subjects under each of the three treatment conditions. A course of treatment consisted of 10 sessions extending over a 3-month period. Subjects were mildly overweight female college students (Fig. 9-3).

At the end of treatment, and 8 weeks later, the results of the behavior modification groups were superior not only to those of the deferred-treatment controls, but also to those of the placebo control groups (Fig. 9-3). The "social pressure" group participated in 20-minute sessions based upon those of TOPS (Take Off Pounds Sensibly) (7). The sessions included a weigh-in, verbal praise for weight loss, encouragement for failure to lose weight, and the wearing of such artifacts as a star for weight loss, a sign in

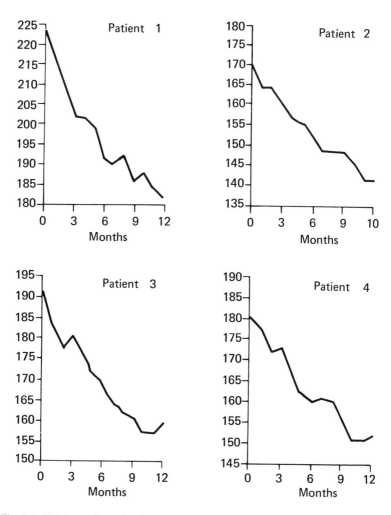

Fig. 9-1. Weight profiles of eight women undergoing behavior therapy for obesity. *A*, Patients 1–4. *B*, Patients 5-8.

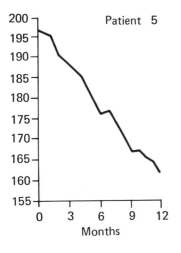

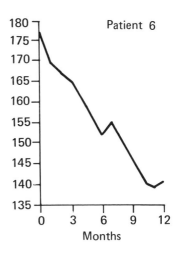

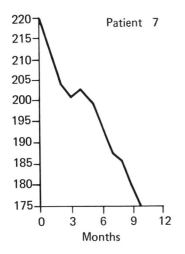

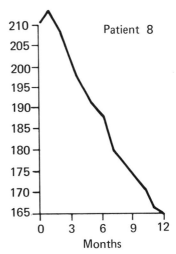

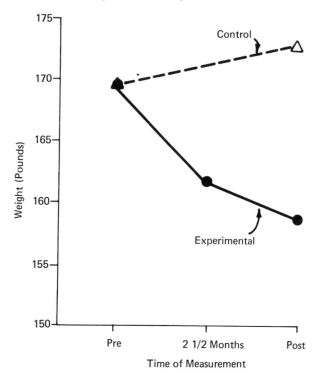

Fig. 9-2. Mean weights for experimental and control subjects.

the form of a pig for weight gain, and sign reading "turtle" for no change in weight. The purpose of this technique was to foster a high positive expectation for losing weight and to develop and use social pressure to help subjects reduce.

The purpose of the "nonspecific therapy" group was to control for the effects of nonspecific factors such as increased attention, faith, expectation of relief, and presentation of a treatment rationale. The rationale was that the treatment should help subjects to develop insight into the "real and not readily recognizable underlying reasons" for their behavior and to discover the "unconscious motives" underlying their personality make-up. Each subject was told that as she obtained insight and better understanding of the "real motives and forces" operating within her personality, she would find it easier to lose weight.

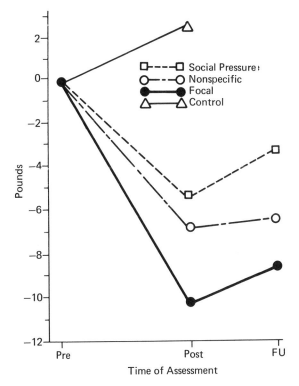

Fig. 9-3. Mean weight loss of the focal (behavioral) treatment group, two alternative treatment control groups, and the no-treatment control group. Treatment lasted 3 months and follow-up (*FU*) occurred 8 weeks later.

The next step in this fascinating development was taken by Richard Hagen (2), who accepted Wollersheim's finding that behavior modification is the most effective method for the treatment of obesity. He turned his attention to answering a resulting question: Were Wollersheim's results due only to the specific behavioral techniques, or were they dependent also upon the interpersonal influence of the therapist? What he proposed, in short, was therapy without a therapist.

Hagen's experimental design was similar to that of Wollersheim. The various treatment groups were compared with each other and with a deferred-treatment control group: (1) behavior modification, 18 subjects; (2) bibliotherapy (use of a written manual), 18 subjects; (3) group and bibliotherapy combined, 18 subjects; (4) deferred-treatment control, 35 subjects.

Hagen's bibliotherapy consisted of a manual, quite similar to that used by the therapists in carrying out behavior modification. It was, however, converted into a programmed text which was mailed weekly to the patients in the bibliotherapy treatment group. They carried out the various exercises, filled out forms just as did the patients in the more traditional behavior therapy group, and then mailed them back for comments.

The 90 subjects in the study were mildly overweight female college students who were randomly assigned to one of the four experimental groups. Three therapists treated six subjects each in group therapy and in the combined therapy conditions. Ten treatment sessions were held over a 3-month period. The most important finding (Fig. 9-4) is that there was no difference in the amount of weight lost by patients whose treatment was accomplished through the manual and those whose treatment was carried out by a therapist. Each group lost an average of 12 lb. The patients who were treated by a combination of bibliotherapy and group treatment lost slightly more weight, as might be expected, but this difference did not reach statistical significance.

Hagen's study shows that it is possible to treat obesity by means of a manual that embodies behavioral principles, and that this treatment is apparently as effective as one that utilizes therapists. I think that this study is going to have a profound effect upon our understanding of psychotherapy. For the greatest effect of any psychotherapy is usually contributed by the therapist himself. The size of this effect of the therapist makes it particularly difficult to distinguish between the substantive differences in various forms of psychotherapy. Hagen's achievement may mean that we can now design studies which can compare substantive differences in psychotherapeutic techniques. Such studies may be able to tell us far more than any yet carried out regarding the efficacy of various approaches.

Another interesting facet of Hagen's study is that the weight losses are considerably larger than those in Wollershim's study. Even the deferred-treatment control groups differed: Wollersheim's subjects gained 2 lb, and Hagen's subjects lost 2 lb. After a great deal of pondering over these results, and talking with both Wollersheim and Hagen, the three of us arrived at an appealing explanation of these differences: Wollersheim's study was carried out in the fall, Hagen's in the spring. The differences in weight apparently arose from differences in the attitude of young women

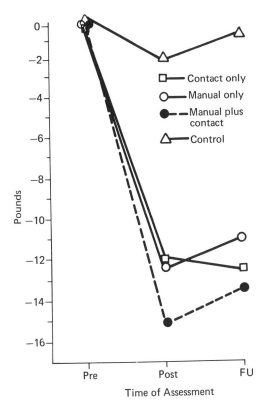

Fig. 9-4. Mean weight loss of three treatment groups and of the no-treatment control group. The former lost significantly more weight than the latter, but there was no significant difference in weight loss between the three treatment groups. Treatment lasted 3 months and follow-up occurred 1 month later.

facing Thanksgiving, Christmas, and New Year's feasts from those of other young women highly motivated to look their best in bathing suits.

The three studies which followed Stuart's original one dealt with rather special patient populations—mildly overweight college women. But what happens to the moderate to severely overweight persons who come to the family doctor for help? Can behavior modification help them? A group of us took a look at the behavioral approach to patients who averaged 80% overweight. We also made an attempt to eliminate some of the bias which may have crept into the earlier studies, for the therapists may have been biased in favor of behavior modification and may well have tried harder with the patients in behavior therapy than with those in the alternate treatment groups. We approached this problem by using different therapists for the different treatment modalities and securing therapists who were frankly biased in favor of the technique they used. Our behavior modifiers were a male experimental psychologist with a strong background in learning theory and a female research technician. Neither had carried out therapy before. Our control groups, on the other hand, were treated by an experienced clinician, Sydnor Penick, with extensive experience in the treatment of obesity. He is a skilled therapist, personable, likable, and dynamic, who knows a great deal about obesity. Dr. Penick's cotherapist was his research nurse who had worked with him in the treatment of obesity over a period of years. They used their traditional methods of supportive psychotherapy, instruction in dieting and nutrition, and, upon demand, appetite suppressants (4). Clearly, if skill and experience were to determine the outcome of this study, behavior modification would lose.

Figure 9-5 shows that the behavior modification groups did better. In each cohort, the median weight loss fo;the behavior modification group was greater than that for the control group—24 lb vs 18 lb for the first cohort; 13 lb vs 11 lb for the second.

The results of treatment of the two cohorts and the persisting effect 1 year after the end of treatment are given in Table 9-1. Over half of the patients in the behavior modification group lost more than 20 lb, and each of these had maintained her weight loss 1 year later.

Now, just what is done in the behavior modification of obesity? What is this new method that seems ready to enter our clinical practice? A thorough account is given in the recent book by Stuart and Davis, "Slim Chance in a Fat World" (6).

Four general principles were utilized in our program: (1) description of behavior to be controlled; (2) modification and control of discriminative stimuli governing eating; (3) development of techniques to control the act of eating; (4) prompt reinforcement of behaviors that delay or control eating.

Description of the Behavior To Be Controlled

The patients were asked to keep daily records of the amount, time, and circumstances of their eating. The immediate results of this time-

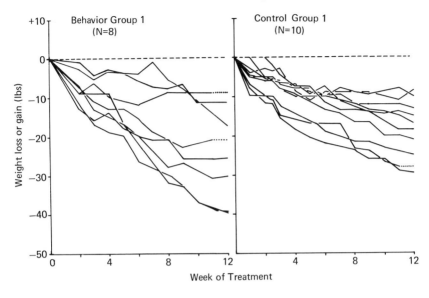

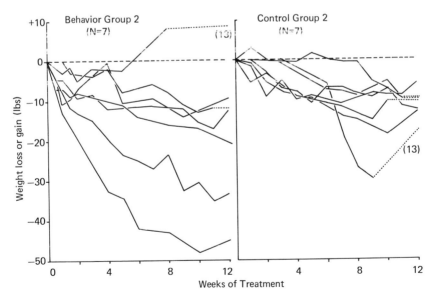

Fig. 9-5. Weight changes of patients in the two cohorts. Dotted lines represent interpolated data based upon weights obtained during follow-up. *A*, Cohort 1. *B*, Cohort 2.

Table 9-1.   Results of Treatment at University of Pennsylvania

	Percent of groups losing specified amounts of weight				
	Behavior modification groups (No. =15)		Control therapy groups (No. =17)		Average in medical literature at end of treatment (8)
Weight loss (lb)	After treatment	1-yr follow-up	After treatment	1-yr follow-up	
>40	13	33	0	12	5
>30	33	40	0	29	—
>20	53	53	24	47	25

consuming and inconvenient procedure were grumbling and complaints. Eventually, however, each patient reluctantly acknowledged that keeping these records had proved very helpful, particularly in increasing his awareness of how much he ate, the speed with which he ate, and the large variety of environmental and psychological situations associated with eating. For example, after 2 weeks of record-keeping, a 30-year-old housewife reported that, for the first time in her life, she recognized that anger stimulated her eating. Accordingly, whenever she began to get angry, she left the kitchen and wrote down how she felt, thereby decreasing her anger and aborting her eating.

Modification and Control of the Discriminative Stimuli Governing Eating

Most of the patients reported that their eating took place in a wide variety of places at many different times during the day. It was postulated that these times and places had become so-called discriminative stimuli signaling eating. The concept of a discriminative stimulus derives from the animal laboratory, where such stimuli as the flashing of a light or sounding of a tone may signal to an animal that pressing a lever will produce food pellets or other reward. Since the reinforcer never occurs without the discriminative stimulus, in the language of learning theory, the stimuli come to "control" various forms of behavior. In an effort to decrease the potency of the discriminative stimuli that controlled their eating, patients were encouraged to confine eating, including snacking, to one place. To avoid disrupting domestic routines, this place was usually the kitchen. Further efforts to control discriminative stimuli included using distinctive table settings, perhaps an unusually colored place mat and napkins. In addition, patients were encouraged to make eating a pure experience, unaccompanied by other activity such as reading, watching television, or arguing with their families.

Development of Techniques To Control the Act of Eating

Specific techniques were utilized to help patients decrease their speed of eating, to become aware of all the components of the eating process, and to gain control over these components. Exercises included counting each mouthful of food eaten during a meal, placing utensils on the plate after every third mouthful until that mouthful was chewed and swallowed, and introducing a 2-min interruption of the meal.

Prompt Reinforcement of Behaviors That Delay or Control Eating

A reinforcement schedule, using a point system, was devised for control of eating behavior. Exercise of the suggested control procedures during a meal earned a certain number of points. These points were converted into money, which was brought to the next meeting and donated to the group. At the beginning of the program, the groups decided how the money should be used, and they chose highly altruistic uses. Each week one group donated its savings to the Salvation Army and another to a needy friend of one of the members, a widow with 14 children.

REFERENCES

1. Ferster CB, Nurnberger JI, Levitt EB: The control of eating. J Mathetics 1:87-109, 1962
2. Hagen RL: Group Therapy Versus Bibliotherapy in Weight Reudction. Thesis. Champaign, Univ Illinois, 1969
3. Harris MB: Self-directed program for weight control: A pilot study. J Abnorm Psychol 74:263-270, 1969
4. Penick, SB, Filion R, Fox S, and Stunbard AJ: Behavior modification in treatment of obesity. Psychosom Med 33:49-55, 1971
5. Stuart RB: Behavioral control of overeating. Behav Res Ther 5:357-365, 1967

6. Stuart RB, Davis B: Slim Chance in a Fat World: Behavioral Control of Obesity. Champaign, Ill, Research Press, 1971

7. Stunkard AJ, Levine H, and Fox S: The management of obesity: Patient self-help and medical treatment. Arch Intern Med 125:1067-1072, 1970

8. Stunkard AJ, McLaren-Hume M: The results of treatment for obesity. Arch Intern Med 103: 79-85, 1959

9. Wollersheim JP: The effectiveness of group therapy based upon learning principles in the treatment of overweight women. J Abnorm Psychol 76:462-474, 1970

Pharmacological Approach to the Treatment of Obesity

10

GEORGE A. BRAY

Obesity is a problem of energy balance. In its final analysis too many calories are ingested relative to the body needs. Thus any form of treatment must be aimed at altering the balance between caloric intake and output. One classification of several approaches that have been used to treat obesity is shown in Table 10-1. The discussion to follow will focus on the use of pharmacologic agents. The first assumption underlying this discussion is my belief that the ultimate solution to the treatment of patients who are substantially overweight—*i.e.,* more than 20%—lies in some form of drug therapy. Although none of the currently available agents provide this solution, it is hoped that the pharmaceutical industry will come up with more effective techniques for dealing with this problem. Since obesity is a chronic symptom, any effective treatment must be

These studies were supported by Grants RR 00425, RR 52, and AM 15165 from the National Institutes of Health.

117

Table 10-1. Classification of Approaches to Treating Obesity

Approach	Current methods
Decrease caloric intake	Total starvation Caloric restriction Anorectic drugs

Enhance caloric output
    Accelerate metabolism
    Malabsorption (fecal)
    Urinary ketones
	Thyroid hormones
	Jejunoileal bypass
	Ketogenic diet

long-term. Therapy can't stop when a patient reaches his goal. If this happens, he will go back to eating the way he ate before starting therapy and weight will reaccumulate. The failure of almost all approaches to the treatment of "the obesities" is that they are short-term. Most physicians can get people to lose some weight, but the real problem is how to keep them reduced. My second assumption is that obesity is a heterogeneous entity. It has both genetic and environmental influences (see Chapt. 5). Since the etiology of most obesity is unknown, the treatment must be largely empirical.

There are several approaches to dealing with the imbalance between caloric intake and expenditure. The first is to decrease food intake by voluntary means. For many patients this is difficult, and the amphetamines and their derivative have been used as an aid in decreasing appetite. There are at present a large number of anorectic drugs related chemically to amphetamines which are available to physicians (Table 10-2). The physiologic effects of four agents that were carefully studied (36, 45) showed that they all raised blood pressure and heart rate, increased respiration, elevated body temperature to a small degree, and caused midryasis. Germane to the present discussion was the finding that they all reduced food intake, which has served as the basis for their use in the therapy of obesity (25). The anorexia seen with amphetamine and some of its congeners could result from interaction of this drug with the central nervous system or by modification of some peripheral metabolic process(es). In recent studies from the Rockefellar University amphetamines were administered directly into the feeding and satiety centers in the hypothalamus of experimental animals. Using this experimental technique, Leibowitz (32) showed that amphetamines decreased food intake when applied directly to the brain, suggesting that their primary action may be on the hypothalamus.

The effectiveness of amphetamines in treating people who are overweight depends upon one's definition of "effectiveness." There is unequivical evidence that in the short term most of the agents on the market will produce greater weight loss than a placebo (12, 18, 33, 44, 46, 49). In a double-blind study (44) comparing a placebo tablet with three active agents, there was a significantly greater weight loss over the 12 weeks' period with each drug than with the placebo (Table 10-3). The weakness of almost all such studies is that treatment period stops at 12 weeks or less. Forty (18) and 24 weeks are the longest duration of continuous treatment that I can find in the literature. Both suffer from the high rate at which patients dropped out of the study. At the end of 24 weeks less than 20% of those who started remained in the program (33).

Although amphetamines will produce weight loss that is greater than placebo, the effects appear to be of short duration. The problem of habituation and drug abuse is a major drawback to these agents. There appear to be major differences, however, in the potential for abuse. On one hand are such widely used and abused drugs as D-amphetamine and methamphetamine and at the other extreme is fenfluramine (Pondimin) with a very low potential for abuse (15). The degree of abuse among obese patients who receive these drugs for treatment is unclear and must await further study.

Biguanides are a second group of drugs which might be classified as anorectic agents. The results of a 2-year study comparing phenformin (DBI) and a sulfonylurea in diabetic patients showed a significant weight loss which was produced and maintained in the group treated with phenformin but did not occur in the group receiving the sulfonylurea. This difference between agents is interesting and provocative and may provide some additional approaches to treating obesity. Glucose tolerance improved in the patients treated with either sulfonylurea or phenformin but not in those treated with placebo. The effects of these drugs on insulin release, however, was very different. With the sulfonylurea, the improved glucose tolerance probably results from the increased levels of insulin. With phenformin glucose tolerance improved, but the secretion of insulin in response to glucose was less than before treatment. Since insulin treatment can enhance food intake in experimental animals, it is conceivable that the reduction in insulin levels during treatment with

Table 10-2: Drugs Used for Control of Appetite

Probable BNDD schedule[a]	Generic name	Trade name	Chemical structure	Usual single dose (mg)
Schedule II	D-Amphetamine	Many	phenyl–CH_2–CH(CH_3)–NH_2	5–15
	Methamphetamine	Many	phenyl–CH_2–CH(CH_3)–NH_2–CH_3	2.5–5.0
Schedule III	Benzphetamine	Didrex	phenyl–CH_2–CH(CH_3)–N(CH_3)–CH_2–phenyl	50
	Phentermine	Ionamin	phenyl–CH_2–C(CH_3)(CH_3)–NH_2	15,30
	Chlorphentermine	Pre-Sate	Cl–phenyl–CH_2–C(CH_3)(CH_3)–NH_2	65
	Diethylpropion	Tenuate Tepanil	phenyl–C(=O)–CH(CH_3)–N(C_2H_5)(C_2H_5)	25–75

	Phenmetrazine	Preludin	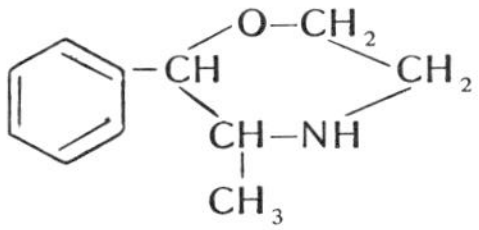	25
	Phendimetrazine	Dietrol Plegine	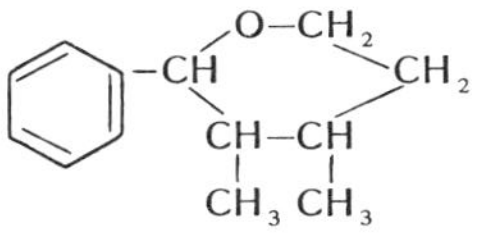	35
	Mazindol	Sanorex	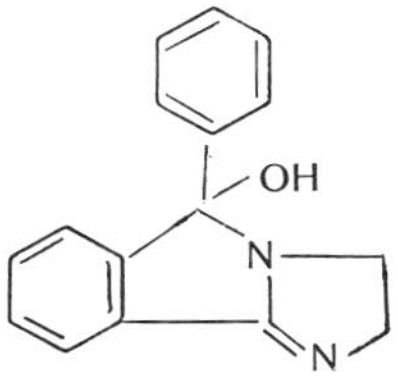	1-2
	Clortermine	Voranil	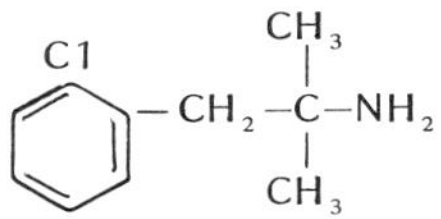	50
Schedule IV	Fenfluramine	Pondimin	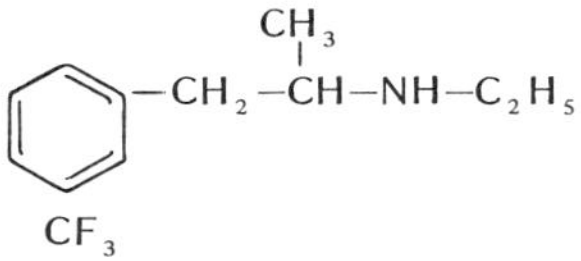	20

[a]Probable scheduling as suggested in Wall Street Journal.

Table 10-3.   Effects of Placebo and Three Drugs on Body Weight Loss During 12
              Weeks of Treatment

Agent	Weight loss (lb)
Placebo	0.9
Phenmetrazine	8.8^a
D-Amphetamine	7.9^a
Benzphetamine	6.5^a

Results obtained in eight subjects randomly distributed in double-blind trial (44).

[a] P <0.01 compared to placebo group.

phenformin may have reduced the stimulating effect of insulin on food intake.

Digitalis has been used in the past for the treatment of obesity. Its anorectic effects result from the narrow tolerance between the therapeutic and toxic effects of this drug. The fatal consequence to patients who had received it in conjunction with other medications makes it unwarranted in treating obesity (27). The American Society of Bariatric Physicians has conducted a double-blind study of digitalis and placebo in a group of patients and showed that digitalis did not enhance weight loss. In their opinion, too, there is no place for digitalis in the treatment of obesity. Digitalis should be reserved for the treatment of congestive heart failure.

A second broad approach to the treatment of obesity is to reduce the absorption of food by the gastrointestinal tract. This is the mechanism behind the use of jejunoileal bypass operations (for a detailed discussion of this surgical approach see Chapt. 11). At present there is no satisfactory pharmacologic method to achieve the same end. A reversible pharmacologic technique for producing malabsorption, however, has three obvious advantages: (1) Risks of surgery are avoided, (2) drugs could be withdrawn if needed; and (3) desired effect could be titrated. Cholestyramine, a drug which complexes bile acids and increases fecal loss of fat has been tried for this purpose in obese patients. Unfortunately, it does not produce adequate steatorrhea, and newer approaches are needed.

A third pharmacologic approach to obesity is to increase caloric utilization. Among the potential drugs with this function, thyroid hormone has been the most widely used. For many years there has been conflict and frustration about various methods of treating obesity. One of the major controversies has been about the use of thyroid hormones.

Although the consensus had gradually evolved that thyroid medication had little to offer (14), the issue was resurrected in 1963 by the observations of Gordon *et al.* (23). In that study, the investigators at the University of Wisconsin suggested that a 1330-Cal diet divided into six feedings and supplemented with polyunsaturated fatty acid was more effective in inducing weight loss when supplemented with triiodothyronine and a mercurial diuretic (23). Their observations suffered, however, from the lack of control data on the effects of diet alone.

To investigate this problem further, we repeated their studies on three groups of subjects: Group I received diet alone; Group II received the diet and a mercurial diuretic; Group III received the complete program, including triiodothyronine and the mercurial diuretic. The five patients who received the complete program (Group III) lost significantly more weight than either of the other groups of patients (6) (Table 10-4). This effect of triiodothyronine was clear whether the results were expressed in terms of absolute weight loss or as a percentage of weight lost. These data tended to support the observation of Gordon *et al.* (23) and are in harmony with several other reports suggesting that thyroid hormones tend to potentiate weight loss in obese subjects (1, 2, 5, 13, 17, 24, 26, 29, 30, 35). The mechanism of this effect is not entirely clear, but considerable information is available regarding thyroid function of obese patients and the metabolic effects of treating them with thyroid hormones.

Protein-bound iodine (PBI) has been measured in obese patients with a diversity of results; some authors have reported low values for PBI (51) while others have suggested that the PBI is similar to values in lean individuals (20). Recent studies in our laboratory, measuring thyroxine

Table 10-4. Effect of Triiodothyronine and Mercurial Diuetics on Weight Loss in Obese Patient

		Weight loss	
Group[a]	No. patients	kg	% of initial wt
I	5	4.6 ± 0.5	4.3 ± 0.3
II	5	5.5 ± 0.7	4.45 ± 0.4
III	5	6.4 ± <0.6	6.3 ± 0.5[b]

[a] I, Diet only; II, diet plus mercurial diuretic every 10 days; III, same as Group II plus triiodothyronine increased stepwise to 150 µg/day.

[b] $P < 0.01$ compared to Group I and II.

and triiodothyronine by radioimmunoassay, indicate that obese subjects do not differ from normal (7). Moreover, we could find no significant correlation between body weight and the concentrations of triiodothyronine or thyroxine in the serum. In harmony with these results is the almost uniform observation that the metabolic rate of obese patients, expressed per unit surface area, is within normal limits (4). This fact has been reported for adolescents (39, 40) and adults (9, 28, 38, 40, 41, 54) over a wide range of body weights. In addition, thyroidal uptake of radioactive iodine is normal and can be suppressed normally by exogenous triiodothyronine (7).

There are a few reports suggesting an abnormality in thyroid function in the obese patient. These include the report of Premachandra *et al.* (47), who observed that a small proportion of obese patients have altered serum binding of circulating thyroid hormones. In addition, Nicoloff and Drenick (42) and Rabinowitz and Myerson (48) observed that obese patients may manifest reduced rates of clearance of thyroid hormones from blood. Oddie *et al.* (43) also suggest that there is a tendency to decreased thyroxine turnover in obesity.

Doses of triiodothyronine above 100 μg/day consistently increase metabolic rate (7). The effect is small but readily measured. However, data from a number of laboratories suggest that doses of T_3 in excess of 150 μg/day will produce untoward symptoms in a few patients (7, 11, 26). To evaluate the effects of T_3 further, we have treated 12 obese patients with T_3, 225 μg/day for 1 month. All patients, however, showed objective alterations in metabolism, including slight tachycardia and increased concentrations of plasma tyrosine (7). These data indicate that for evaluating unwanted side effects, clinical criteria are insensitive to the metabolic consequences of treatment with thyroid hormones in some obese patients.

Thyroid hormones can increase nitrogen excretion (7, 38). Within the first few days after administration of exogenous thyroid hormone, there is loss of nitrogen and a negative nitrogen balance. This effect persists for at least 30 days, although it reaches its peak within the first 10 days. Whether nitrogen balance returns to normal on small doses of thyroid hormone and how long this takes is presently unknown. Two recent studies indicate that the loss of nitrogen can be prevented. In one study, anabolic steroids and growth hormone were used to prevent the loss of nitrogen induced by treatment with triiodothyronine with no decrease in oxygen consumption

(8). In the other report the loss of nitrogen was prevented in increasing the dietary intake of protein (31).

The cardiac effects of thyroid hormone have been widely studied in experimental and clinical states, but the mechanism of these effects is still not clearly established. In obese patients triiodothyronine will increase heart rate (Fig. 10-1), and the effect is probably dependent on dosage. In experimental animals, thyroid hormones also increase the size of the heart, and this may also happen in humans (52).

Thyroid hormones can also modify the secretion of growth hormone in obesity. This has been shown using arginine, one of several provocative stimuli for increasing the circulating concentration of growth hormone in

Fig. 10-1. Effect of triiodothyronine (T_3) or placebo on weight loss and heart rate Twelve patients were treated for 1 month with T_3 (225 μg/day) and 1 month with placebo. Weight loss was significantly greater with T_3 than with placebo. Heart rate was significantly increased by 6 beats per minute.

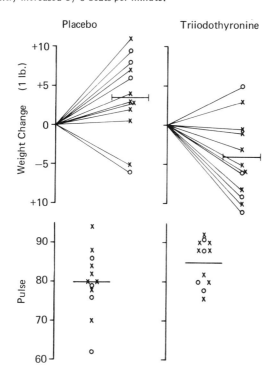

normal subjects. When arginine is infused into obese patients, the rise in growth hormone concentration is markedly reduced. In contrast, after 14-21 days of pretreatment with triiodothyronine (200 μg/day), arginine evokes a much greater release of growth hormone than before treatment (34). Thyroid hormones can also modify the release of free fatty acids (FFA) (37). According to Mautalen and Smith (47), the epinephrine-induced release of FFA is significantly less in obese patients than in normal subjects although other groups have not found this (21). After pretreatment with triiodothyronine (but allegedly not with thyroxine), the rise in FFA after epinephrine is augmented.

Finally, thyroid hormones stimulate the metabolism of glycerol-3-phosphate in adipose tissue. The activity of the mitochondrial glycerophosphate oxidase, which converts glycerol-3-phosphate to dihydroxyacetone phosphate, is less in obese patients than in lean subjects (16). The activity of this enzyme can be increased by a high caloric diet or by pretreatment with triiodothyronine (5). This effect of T_3 has been observed in adipose tissue of human subjects as well as experimental animals (50).

From the above discussion, it is clear that thyroid hormones induce a number of changes in obese patients which will tend to enhance their weight loss. Although some of these effects are desirable, others are not and have been used as arguments against the safety of thyroid hormone in the treatment of obesity. One useful effect is the stimulation of oxygen consumption with increased utilization of endogenous fuel. Undesirable is the acceleration of protein catabolism and increased nitrogen excretion. (3) Although approximately two-thirds of the extra calories expended as a result of treatment with T_3 occur from catabolism of fat (7), the majority of the weight loss results from breakdown of protein by treatment with triiodothyronine.[1] This fact is frequently used as an argument against treating obese patients with these hormones. Recent studies by Lamki *et al.*

[1] This difference is easy to understand if one thinks about the caloric density of adipose tissue vs. lean body mass. Adipose tissue is approximately 15% water and thus contains about 7.5 Cal/g wet tissue. In contrast, lean body tissue is approximately three-quarters water with only one-quarter being energy-producing protein. Thus, the caloric density of hydrated lean body tissue is approximately 1.5 Cal/g. Thus, it takes 5 g lean tissue to produce as many calories as 1 g fat. With one-quarter of the calories coming from metabolism of lean body tissue, one would expect that over one-half of the weight would come primarily from the loss of intracellular water which occurs when protein is catabolized.

(31), however, have suggested that increasing the protein content of the diet can overcome this catabolic effect. Thus, losses of nitrogen do not seem to provide a serious drawback to the safety of thyroid hormones in obesity.

A more potentially dangerous problem is the effect of thyroid hormone administration on cardiac function. These effects include modification of the chronotropic and inotropic properties of cardiac muscle. Although the mechanism(s) for these effects is not known, it is clear that treatment with thyroid hormones in experimental animals, and probably in man, will increase the mass of the heart (52). Since obesity itself increases the weight of the heart (10), the added cardiac load imposed by treatment with thyroid hormones could be detrimental. Indeed, the deleterious cardiac effects of dextrothyroxine observed when this agent is used to lower serum lipids in patients with atherosclerosis have led to its withdrawal from the trial of agents used in the treatment of patients with coronary artery disease (53).

Finally, the beneficial effects, if any, of treatment of obese patients with thyroid hormones must be evaluated by their long-term effectiveness. Unfortunately, there are few careful long-term follow-up studies which provide this information. In most studies using diet as the predominant mode of treatment, 25% of the patients will achieve and maintain a weight loss of 20 lbs or more for 1 year. However, less than 10% will maintain a 40-lb weight loss for 1 year. In one long-term study 27 out of 33 patients were traced for 14 years after an initial dietary treatment. Five out of the 27 had maintained their initial weight loss for the entire periods, but the others had regained as much as or more than they had lost (55). Thus, to be effective, thyroid hormone would have to produce a long-term decrease in body weight which is greater than that produced by diet alone. In one study, Asher and Dietz (2) evaluated weight loss in a program involving thyroid hormone and amphetamines. They claimed that 10% achieved a weight loss of 40 lbs or more and that 38% had a weight loss of more than 20 lbs. Unfortunately, the follow-up in this study was less than 1 year, and it is not clear that their results were significantly greater than those achieved with careful dietary management. At least two studies have indicated that small dosages of thyroid hormones (3 grains of USP thyroid or 75 μg of triiodothyronine) can potentiate the action of amphetamine (17, 29). These studies, too, suffer from the short duration of patient follow-up. In one long-term study, Glennon (19) noted that patients treated with triiodothyronine had a low rate of long-term success. Only 12.5% of the group maintained a significant weight loss after more than a year and only one patient in this group of nearly 200 approached ideal body weight. Similarly discouraging data have been obtained by Goodman (22) in a comparison of triiodothyronine and placebo. There is thus no convincing evidence that thyroid hormone produce a more significant and sustained weight loss than carefully administered management using diet as the sole modality of treatment.

In spite of these discouraging results, hope springs eternal. It is this investigator's belief that new and more effective drugs for the long-term treatment of obesity will become available in the future. Such agents will better enable the physician concerned with obesity to treat his patients successfully.

REFERENCES

1. Adlersberg D, Mayer E: Results of prolonged medical treatment of obesity with diet alone, diet and thyroid preparations and diet and amphetamine. J Clin Endocrinol Metab 9:275-284, 1949

2. Asher WL, Dietz RE: Effectiveness of weight reduction involving "diet pills." Curr Ther Res 14:510-524, 1972

3. Ball MF, Kyle LH, Canary JJ: Comparative effects of caloric restriction and metabolic acceleration of body composition in obesity. J Clin Endocrinol Metab 27:273-278, 1967

4. Boothby WM, Sandiford I: Summary of the basal metabolism data on basal metabolic rate. J Biol Chem 54:783-804, 1922

5. Bray GA: The effect of diet and triiodothyronine on the activity of sn-glycerol-3-phosphate dehydrogenase and on the metabolism of glucose and pyruvate by adipose tissue of obese patients. J Clin Invest 48: 1413-1422, 1969

6. Bray GA: The myth of diet in the management of obesity. Am J Clin Nutr 23:1141-1148, 1970

7. Bray GA, Melvin KEW, Chopra IF: The effect of triiodothyronine on some metabolic responses of obese patients. Am J Clin Nutr 26:715-721, 1973

8. Bray GA, Raben MS, Londono J, Gallagher TF Jr: Effects of triiodothyronine, growth hormone and anabolic steroids on nitrogen excretion and oxygen consumption of obese patients. J Clin Endocrinol Metab 33:293-300, 1971

9. Bray GA, Schwartz M, Rozin R, Lister J: Relationships between oxygen consumption and body composition of obese patients. Metabolism 19:418-429, 1970

10. Chiang BN, Perlman LV, Epstein FH: Overweight and hypertension: A review. Circulation 39:403-421, 1969

11. Cornman D, Alexander F: Effects of 1-triiodothyronine alone in the treatment of obesity (abstr). Fed Proc 24:189, 1965

12. Diethylpropion, an Appetite Suppressant. The Medical Letter 13(No 25):101-105, 1971

13. Drenick DJ, Fisler JL: Prevention of recurrent weight gain with large doses of thyroid hormones. Curr Ther Res 12:570-576, 1970

14. Editorial. JAMA 204:328, 1969

15. Fenfluramine. The Medical Letter. 15:(8) 33-34 April 13, 1972

16. Galton DJ, Bray GA: Metabolism of α-glycerol phosphate in human adipose tissue in obesity. J Clin Endocrinol Metab 27:1573-1580, 1967

17. Gelvin EP, Kenigsberg S, Boyd LJ: Results of addition of liothyronine to a weight-reducing regimen. JAMA 170:1507-1512, 1959

18. Gelvin EP, McGavack TH: Dexedrine and weight reduction. NY State J Med 49:279-282, 1949

19. Glennon JA: Weight reduction—an enigma. Arch Intern Med 118:1-2, 1966

20. Glennon JA, Brech WJ: Serum protein bound iodine in obesity. J Clin Endocrinol Metab 25:1673-1674, 1965

21. Glennon JA, Brech WJ, Gordon ES: Evaluation of an epinephrine test in obesity. Metabolism 14:1240-1242, 1965

22. Goodman NG: Triiodothyronine and placebo in the treatment of obesity. Med Ann DC 38:658-662, 1969

23. Gordon ES, Goldberg M, Chosy GJ: A new concept in the treatment of obesity. JAMA 186:156-166, 1963

24. Gwinup G, Poucher R: A controlled study of thyroid analogs in the therapy of obesity, Am J Med Sci 254:416-420, 1967

25. Harris SC, Ivy AC, Searle LM: The mechanism of amphetamine-induced loss of weight: A consideration of the theory of hunger and appetite. JAMA 134:1468-1475, 1947

26. Hollingsworth DR, Amatruda TT Jr, Scheig R: Quantitative and qualitative effects of 1-triiodothyronine in massive obesity. Metabolism 19:934-945, 1970

27. Jelliffe RW, Hill D, Tatter D *et al:* Death from weight control pills. JAMA 208:1843-1847, 1969

28. Johnston LC, Bernstein LM: Body composition and oxygen consumption of overweight, normal and underweight women. J Lab Clin Med 45:109-118, 1955

29. Kaplan NM, Jose A: Thyroid as an adjuvant to amphetamine therapy of obesity: A controlled double-blind study. Am J Med Sci 260:105-111, 1970

30. Kneebone GM: Drug therapy: An effective treatment of obesity in childhood. Med J Aust 2:663-665, 1968

31. Lamki L, Ezrin C, Koven I, Steiner G: L-Thyroxine in the treatment of obesity with no increase in loss of lean body mass. Metabolism 22:611-622, 1973

32. Leibowitz SF: Reciprocal hunger-regulating circuits involving alpha- and beta-adrenergic receptors located respectively, in the ventromedial and lateral hypothalamus. Proc Nat Acad Sci 67:1063-1070, 1970

33. Le Riche WH, Csima A: A long-acting appetite suppressant drug studied for 24 weeks in both continuous and sequential administration. Can Med Assoc J 97:1016-1020, 1967

34. Londono J, Gallagher TF Jr, Bray GA: Effect of weight reduction, triiodothyronine and diethylstilbestrol on growth hormone in obesity. Metabolism 18:986-992, 1969

35. Lyon DM, Dunlop DM: The treatment of obesity. A comparison of the effects of diet and of thyroid extract. Quart J Med 1:331-352, 1932

36. Martin WR, Sloan JW, Sapira JD, Jasinski DR: Physiologic, subjective and behavioral effects of amphetamine, methamphetamine, ephedrine, phenmetrazine and methylphenidate in man. Clin Pharmacol Ther 12:245-258, 1971

37. Mautalen C, Smith RW Jr: Effects of triiodothyronine and thyroxin on the lipolytic action of epinephrine in markedly obese subjects. Am J Clin Nutr 16:363-369, 1965

38. Means JH: The basal metabolism in obesity. Arch Intern Med 17:704, 1916

39. Mossberg HO: Obesity in children: A clinical-prognostical investigation. Acta Pediatr 35(Suppl 2):1-122, 1948

40. Nelson RA, Anderson LF, Gastineau CF, Hayles AB, Stamnes CL: Physiology and natural history of obesity. JAMA 223:627-630, 1973

41. Newburgh LH: Obesity. I. Energy metabolism. Physiol Rev 24:18-31, 1944

42. Nicoloff JT, Drenick EJ: Altered peripheral thyroxine metabolism in severe obesity. Clin Res 14:148, 1966

43. Oddie TH, Mead JH Jr, Fisher DA: An analysis of published data on thyroxin turnover in human subjects. J Endocrinol Metab 26:425-436, 1966

44. Patel N, Mock DC Jr, Hagans JA: Comparison of benzphetamine, phenmetrazine, d-amphetamine, and placebo. Clin Pharmacol Ther 4:330-333, 1963

45. Pinter, EJ, Pattee CJ: Fat-mobilizing action of amphetamine. J Clin Invest 47:394-402, 1968

46. Poindexter A: Appetite suppressant drugs: A controlled clinical comparison of benzphetamine. Phenmetrazine, d-amphetamine and placebo. Curr Ther Res 2:354-363, 1960

47. Premachandra BH, Perlstein IB, Blumenthal HT: Thyroid auto-immunity, thyroxine transport, and angiopathy in human obesity in Physiopathology of Adipose Tissue. Edited by J Vague and RM Denton. Amsterdam, Excerpta Medica, 1969, pp 289-301.

48. Rabinowitz JL, Myerson RM: The effects of triiodothyrone on some metabolic parameters of obese individuals. Blood ^{14}C-glucose replacement rate, respiratory ^{14}CO$_2$, the pentose cycle, the biological half-life of T$_3$ and the concentration of T$_3$ in adipose tissue. Metabolism 16:68-75, 1967

49. Resnick M, Joubert L: A double-blind evaluation of an anorexiant, a placebo and diet alone in obese subjects. Can Med Assoc J 97:1011-1015, 1967

50. Rivlin RA, Menedez C, Langdon RG: Biochemical similarities between hypothyroidism and riboflavin deficiency. Endocrinology 83:461-469, 1968

51. Scriba PC, Richter J, Horn K, Breckebans J, Schwarz K: Zur frage der Schilddrusenfunktion bei Adipositas. Klin Wochenschr 45:323-324, 1967

52. Staffurth JS, Morrison NDW: Heart size in thyrotoxicosis. Postgrad Med J 44:885-890, 1968

53. Stamler J: The coronary drug project: Findings leading to further modifications of its protocol with respect to dextrothyroxine. JAMA 220:996-1008, 1972

54. White RI Jr, Alexander JK: Body oxygen consumption and pulmonary ventilation in obese subjects. J Appl Physiol 20:197-210, 1965

55. Sohar E, Sneh E: Follow-up of obese patients: 14 years after a successful reducing diet. Am J Clin Nutr 26: 845-848, 1973

Jejunoileal Bypass Surgery for Obesity

11

LOREN DeWIND

Operative intervention for obesity was initiated over 15 years ago (4) and has been used by several groups (1-3, 5-7). The indications for jejunoileal bypass surgery in the treatment of obesity are as follows.

Weight more than 100 lb over standard for height, sex, and age
Failure of other forms of treatment
Presence of one or more of the following:
    Hypertension
    Pickwickian syndrome
    Abnormal glucose tolerance
    Menstrual dyscrasias
    Infertility
    Degenerative arthritis of hips, knees, or feet
    Frank diabetes mellitus
    Hyperlipidemia
Stable adult life pattern
Acceptance of expected hazards

Agreement to undergo needed revision
Availability of the following:
    Experienced team of internist and surgeon
    Good laboratory and intensive care facilities

The patient with morbid obesity is defined as an individual who is more than 100 lb above ideal weight. To be considered for this procedure such a patient should have a stable, adult life pattern. Living with an operation of this type requires a high degree of cooperation from the patient. We expect people to understand the hazards of the operation and agree to undergo needed surgical revision if this should become necessary.

When we undertook to perform jejunoileal bypass for obesity, we reasoned that perhaps it would be possible to induce loss of weight by a drastic surgical method and when the patient had achieved adequate weight loss, he would be able to maintain it after the shunt had been taken down. The jejunum was transected 15 in. from the ligament of Treitz and implanted directly into the transverse colon, providing a very limited absorptive surface. This procedure did not accomplish what we planned. In most instances, the weight of the first 10 patients undergoing the operation had gone back up to its original level. Although in a few instances we had some degree of success with this approach, it was not a good procedure because of the difficulties and hazards which actually developed.

We have devised a different approach to this operation that has provided a more physiologic absorption pattern and which has been used for more than 150 patients. In the upper intestine, glucose and iron are absorbed as well as many vitamins. Fat and protein, on the other hand, are absorbed farther down. In the ileum, vitamin B_{12} is absorbed and bile acids and bile salts reenter the portal circulation. To take advantage of this knowledge, we decided to leave some ileum in continuity with the jejunum. At first, we anastomized 20 in. of jejunum to 20 in. of ileum. Gradually, we cut the length of the jejunum and ileum, since people with longer shunts did not lose weight very well. At the present time, we connect 14 in. of jejunum to the side of the terminal ileum, 4 in. from the end. We leave the ileocecal valve intact to increase the absorptive surface for water, B_{12} and bile salts by using the terminal ileum and the right colon. The remainder of the intestine is left in situ with the jejunal end closed.

The degree of reflux back into the ileum may be significant, with retrograde flow of 10 or 12 in. being observed. There may be absorption from this intestinal fluid, which may influence the degree of weight loss. In spite of this, most of these patients have lost a gratifying amount of weight. The bypassed intestine remains in a resting state, in contrast to the bowel carrying the intestinal contents, which becomes hypertrophied. In those cases where reanastamosis was necessary, the bowel has completely resumed its normal function within 10-12 days.

We were able to follow up 88 patients for a period of 1 year or more after surgery (3, 4). The mean and median weight loss turned out to be 100 lb at 1 year. People who weigh considerably more than the average for our group usually lose more weight. Those who weigh less than 250 lb will usually not achieve a loss of 100 lb in 1 year. There is greater weight loss in the first 6 months than in the second 6 months. In the third 6-month period, weight loss averages 8 lb/mo. Even in the third year and fourth years this group was still losing at a very small rate.

To learn about longer term weight, we charted a few patients with good follow-up (Fig. 11-1). Two of these patients were approaching 600 lb at the time of surgery. Weight loss was most precipitous initially, then leveled out, and after 5 years, it had stabilized. In no instance has the patient lost more than what we would consider ideal weight loss on the basis of standard height and weight tables. In some instances, we have found that weight gain has occurred very slowly with adaptation to this drastic surgery, but the degree of weight gain has been 10-20 lb, and in one or two instances, more than that, but nobody has returned to his original weight.

Observations that we made on people who have been followed up for a period of 1 year or more showed little change in serum levels of various electrolytes and metabolites. Oral supplements of potassium will keep average potassium levels about what they were before the operation. Some people before the operation had been on diuretics and their mean potassium level was lower than it would be if they had been totally untreated. The blood cholesterol levels dropped in all cases. We have many patients in whom the blood cholesterol level is approximately 70-100 mg/100 ml. The serum protein levels have apparently been maintained quite well. We have not seen significant anemia. Iron absorption is apparently adequate. Glucose tolerance tests improve with weight loss even in frank diabetics, and some even return to the normal range.

The question of what this surgery does to the liver is controversial. There have been some reports pointing out that this is a very hazardous

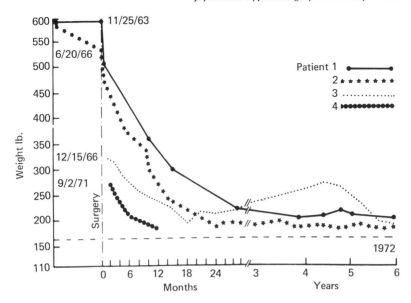

Fig. 11-1. Long- and short-term weight loss patterns after jejunoileal bypass surgery in four patients with morbid obesity.

procedure and should not be performed because of severe, extreme liver damage (6). There has also been information in the literature to the contrary (1, 2). One group studied 10 patients in sequence and attempted to determine the effect of bypass surgery on the liver by biopsy. They found that three appeared worse, three better, two unchanged, and two had no specific changes.

One of our very heavy male patients, 560 lb, lost 350 lb between biopsies. At the time of surgery, there was a lot of fat stored in his liver. At a second operation, 2 years later, the liver appeared entirely normal. There was a little infiltration with lymphocytes, but in general, it was interpreted by our pathologist as being a very normal-appearing liver. Dramatic improvement such as this is not always seen. Biopsy from a girl whose weight was 280 lb showed a fairly normal-looking liver. After the shunt procedure performed by the usual technique, this girl over the next 3 years lost a grand total of 32 lb. At that time a liver biopsy showed a liver that was full of fat. She was eating a normal diet and had no particular complaints.

Another woman lost a lot of weight and was so ill with vomiting and abdominal distress that we were prepared to reconnect her, but a little more study revealed a badly diseased gallbladder. At the time of the gallbladder surgery, a liver biopsy was taken. It was interpreted as showing the effects of severe malnutrition on the liver, with lots of fat storage and fibrosis. After cholecystectomy, she began to improve and is now working as a nurse, maintaining her weight loss and feeling quite comfortable. In another patient, a rather bad-looking liver showed improvement in the fat distribution 4 years later but demonstrated periportal changes. We are fearful that fibrosis may be one of the problems that we will have to cope with. However, some 5 years later, although we have not rebiopsied her liver, clinically this patient does not have any problems.

In one of our longer term follow-ups, a liver biopsy was taken at the time her shunt was established some 12 years ago. She consulted another physician because she had moved from the area and had a revision of the shunt 11 years later. The appearance of the liver some 11 years later was not healthy. There is considerable fat distributed throughout, but the patient has done well clinically. She has had 3 children since the time of the initial surgery and leads a healthy life.

Effects on the liver in jejunocolic shunt are more worrisome. A biopsy made at the time the shunt was taken down in one patient showed marked fatty changes. Six years after the shunt was taken down, this woman regained all of her weight and requested that we do the operation again by the newer technique. The changes in the liver that were present after the first shunt had completely reversed by the time of the second shunt. We wish to emphasize that some of the changes in the liver are totally reversible.

There are other hazards and discomforts from a surgical bypass which a person can expect (Table 11-1). One of the obvious is diarrhea with anal discomfort. Some hazards are predictable and explained to the patient in advance so he will not be too discouraged. For this purpose we use forms similar to those in the Appendix. Hypokalemia can be treated by potassium supplement. The patients learn to tolerate diarrhea because that is the only way the excess food intake gets out of the body. Many people complain of weakness for a period of 6 months or so after surgery. They feel unable to get strong enough to do their usual work. Severe thirst is probably related to the low absorptive surface, with loss of water in liquid stools. Nausea is common. This is quite a variable symptom, but we try to warn patients about it to forestall their disappointment when the friend who referred them says she had no nausea.

Table 11-1. Incidence of Complications After Jejunoileal Bypass in the Treatment of Morbid Obesity

Complication	Incidence (%)
Wound Infection	2
Wound Dehiscence	0.5
Incisional Hernia	3
Intestinal Obstruction or Volvulus	2
Hypokalemia	80
Hypocalcemia	30
Hypoproteinemia	50
Liver Failure	3
Peptic Ulcer	2
Urinary Calculi	10
Arthralgias	15
Renal Failure	3
Severe Nausea and Vomiting	3
Metabolic Acidosis	3

Anal pain and hemorrhoids are quite common. Gout attacks are not frequent, but can be expected occasionally since the blood uric acid goes up in most instances, probably because of tissue breakdown with release of nucleic acids into the circulation. Intussusception may occur but can usually be avoided by proper surgical technique. Patients at first were warned that they might need an operation to correct intussusception of the defunctioned segment of bowel.

Some hazards we really did not anticipate, but we found they were controllable by medical measures. It is unwise for people to drink alcoholic beverages because some of them became highly intoxicated from small amounts of alcohol and developed confused irrational behavior. We have warned all of our patients that they should not consume alcoholic beverages for at least a year after surgery. We also feel that alcohol may impose a severe metabolic load on the liver. Most people cooperate with this restriction. We have found that most obese patients are not alcoholics.

A number of people have developed urinary calculi. We have no satisfactory explanation for this, but there are some interesting speculations about why it happens. The problem is confused by the fact that many people who are obese already have urinary calculi and a number of our patients who have calculi after the shunt tell us that they have had urinary calculi at some time in the past. Pancreatitis is unpredictable, but has occurred in one or two patients, one of whom died from acute pancreatitis. Two or three patients have had bleeding peptic ulcers, which have been treated medically. About 25 patients have had arthralgia, which is usually transient and mild. Macrocytic anemia is very rare and easily treated by vitamin B_{12}, folic acid, or both.

Some hazards are serious and dictate reconnection of the bowel to its original state. If patients develop severe nausea and vomiting that is not controllable with repletion of fluids, electrolytes, and calories, they may rapidly go into a state of protein malnutrition and electrolyte deficiency, which increases the hazard of reoperation. Evidence of deteriorating liver function, as measured by increasing levels of serum enzymes and bilirubin, is an ominous sign and we usually plan reoperation immediately. A few patients have shown advancing renal impairment with hyperchloremic metabolic acidosis. We are not certain what the cause of this is, but think it may be related to damage to the renal tubule because of a severe potassium and bicarbonate deficiency. Hypokalemia which is uncontrollable by oral supplements probably represents an indication for discontinuing the shunt.

Fatalities represent something like 7-8% of our series. This is a gross figure, and I think that with careful analysis the deaths which can be attributed to the procedure itself can be narrowed down considerably. For example, one patient developed breast cancer after surgery. We are not sure whether the surgery had anything to do with the breast cancer or whether weight loss unmasked the cancer. Thromboembolism is a complication of any kind of operation, but we see nothing about the shunt procedure which would make thromboembolism a more frequent complication. Myocardial infarction occurred in two patients before they left the hospital; we proceeded with the operation in one patient, in the hope that we could reverse his heart disease, but, unfortunately, he had an infarct before he left the hospital and died.

We feel that alcoholics with liver failure are not suitable candidates for the shunt. Liver failure itself is still a problem. Until we are able to find out more about why people develop liver failure, we will probably continue to see it in some people. One patient died of myasthenia gravis. One man with renal failure, who had one kidney, developed glomerulonephritis and died.

There are several contraindications to intestinal bypass:

Evidence of serious coronary artery disease
Liver cirrhosis or persistent abnormality of liver enzymes

Advanced age
Emotional immaturity
Hostility to family or physicians
Unwillingness to give up alcohol consumption for at least 1 year
Evident unrealistic expectations

Since the surgery is investigational, we avoid patients over 50 and under 18. Emotional immaturity is a contraindication because of the high degree of cooperation required. Extreme passivity and lack of motivation to lose weight as indicated by failure in the past to make at least some effort to lose is a contraindication. Patients with renal stones must be evaluated carefully before a decision is made to operate.

Patients who are mentally defective or who have an uncooperative home setting should be rejected. If litigation is pending concerning another health problem, it is probably not wise to operate, in view of the new predictable symptoms which may obscure or complicate the picture. The contraindications listed above are relative. Several absolute contraindications exist which include active liver disease, a previous myocardial infarction, previous thromboembolic episodes, a hostile patient and poor renal function.

REFERENCES

1. Berkowitz D: Metabolic changes associated with obesity before and after weight reduction. JAMA 187:399, 1964

2. Juhl E, Christofferson P, Baden H, *et al.:* Hepatic effects of obesity treated with jejunoileal anastomosis. N Engl J Med 285:543-547, 1971

3. Payne JH, DeWind LT: Surgical treatment of obesity. Am J Surg 118:141-147, 1969

4. Payne JH, DeWind LT, Schwab CE, and Kern W: Surgical treatment of morbid obesity: Sixteen years experience. Arch Surg 106:432-437, 1973

5. Scott HW Jr, et al: Jejunoileal shunt in surgical treatment of morbid obesity. Ann Surg 171:770-782, 1970

6. Snodgrass PJ: Obesity, small bowel bypass and liver disease. N Engl J Med 282:870-871, 1970

7. Weismann RE: Surgical palliation of massive and severe obesity. Am J Surg 125:437-446, 1973

8. Westwater JO, Fainer D: Liver impairment in the obese. Gastro-enterology 34:686-693, 1958

Appendix

ADVICE TO PATIENTS UNDERGOING INTESTINAL BYPASS

You have undergone a rather drastic operation designed to limit the absorption of excess calories from your intestinal tract. You will note some or all of the following symptoms:

Diarrhea. This may be severe, with frequent watery bowel movements. It will usually be most severe after your largest meal, and most commonly in the evening and early night-time hours. This is expected and must be tolerated.

Soreness of the rectal area. The passage of chemicals and partly digested food causes this. It is more troublesome to some patients than to others. It gradually gets better unless you have a hemorrhoid problem.

Gassy distention and rumbling. This is variable and unpredictable. It may not occur until several months after surgery.

Loss of appetite. This is common in the early weeks after surgery and usually normal appetite returns in about 6-8 weeks. Your taste for foods may change and you may crave certain things. Within reason this is not harmful.

General physical weakness. This is usually not profound but you may notice lethargy, lack of ambition, sluggishness, and some discouragement.

Pains in the abdomen or side. These may or may not be serious. If more than just passing cramps, they should be reported to the doctor. They may signal a twist in the intestine, or passage of a kidney stone.

Within the first days or weeks after the operation, certain adaptations of the body are necessary and must occur. The most important of these are listed here and form the basis for the recommendations which follow.

—The shortened intestine cannot handle the same quantity of food you normally eat, until it enlarges and stretches after several months.

—The absorption of liquids by the intestine is markedly limited, and most of what you drink will go right through, especially if liquids are taken rapidly.

—The lower intestine is reached by food and liquid far sooner than is normally the case and is shocked by contact with cold or hot liquids (chiefly cold).

—The digestive juices are rapidly poured into the large intestine and produce severe irritation when they reach the rectal area.

—The absorption of certain essential minerals, chiefly potassium, calcium, and sometimes magnesium, as well as bicarbonate, is markedly hampered.

—With lowered food absorption, the body stores of fat are mobilized, and must go to the liver to be metabolized into a form from which the body can derive energy. The liver is under severe stress, as it must store and dispose of this fat load, and change it chemically so the muscles can use it for fuel.

—The kidneys are supplied with far less water than is normal. This results in lower urine output at the same time that large amounts of water run through the intestine. Under these conditions kidney stones may form.

There are other changes occurring in the body, the causes of which are not well understood. It is possible that you may have symptoms or complications not discussed here. It is important that you understand the investigative nature of this procedure and that the medical profession may not yet have all the answers to every problem that may arise.

Recommendations

From our experience we are prepared to make a number of suggestions about diet, daily life pattern, and medication, which should be carefully followed. These directions will help to minimize your discomfort and disability. You must realize, however, that no two cases are alike, and sometimes problems will arise when you do everything right.

—For the first 6 weeks after surgery you should studiously avoid eating or drinking anything colder than room temperature. You will have a craving for cold drinks and very cold foods, such as ice cream. Cold food and drink shocks the newly formed food pathway so it cannot absorb necessary minerals and washes through food elements which should be absorbed.

—You must eat some food every day, even though you have no appetite and feel nauseated. Complete failure to eat stresses the liver severely and prevents replacement of vital minerals and chemicals which cannot be replaced completely even by intravenous therapy.

—You must avoid drinking large quantities of liquid with meals. A little milk on cereal, a cup of soup, and a cup of coffee, tea, or milk are permissible, but in general the meal should be taken quite dry.

—Fluid intake should be spread out over waking hours, but not within a one-half-hour period before or a one-hour period after meals. It would be permissible for example to drink 3 or 4 ounces of water every half hour according to your thirst, but not to drink 1 or 2 quarts at a time every 2 or 3 hours.

—Foods high in potassium should be taken with each meal. Examples are bananas, dried dates, cantaloupe, most fruits, as well as meats. Other high-potassium foods may be found on lists available from your doctor or the Heart Association.

—Alcohol in all forms must be avoided for at least 1 year. The liver metabolism is severely stressed by alcohol, and even small amounts may result in severe liver damage. In addition, alcohol produces effects on the brain which result in bizarre and unpredictable behavior, with danger to self or others.

—You should avoid standing or sitting for long periods in the hot sun, or visiting the desert during the first year. Severe dehydration can occur rapidly from moderate perspiration.

If any of these instructions are not clear, the doctor will be able to clarify them for you by phone or on a regular office visit. If you find a certain technique or way of life that eases some of the problems, we are always happy to learn about it and will pass it along to others.

I hereby certify that I have received a copy of the attached Advice and Recommendations, and that I have read same and agree to follow them to the best of my ability, if selected as a candidate for an intestinal shunt procedure for the control of obesity.

Signed   _____

Date   _____

Witness _____

Index

Page numbers followed by the letter "f" indicate illustrations. Page numbers followed be the letter "n" indicate footnotes. Page numbers followed by the letter "t" indicate tabular material.

74 75 76 77 78 10 9 8 7 6 5 4 3 2 1